ATLAS OF
CANINE AND FELINE
PERIPHERAL BLOOD
SMEARS

ATLAS OF
CANINE AND FELINE
PERIPHERAL BLOOD
SMEARS

First Edition

Amy C. Valenciano, DVM, MS, DACVP
Veterinary Clinical Pathologist
IDEXX Reference Laboratories, Inc.
Dallas, Texas

Rick L. Cowell, DVM, MS, MRCVS, DACVP
Veterinary Clinical Pathologist
IDEXX Laboratories, Inc.
Stillwater, Oklahoma

Theresa E. Rizzi, DVM, DACVP
Clinical Associate Professor
Department of Veterinary Pathobiology
Center for Veterinary Health Sciences
Oklahoma State University
Stillwater, Oklahoma

**Ronald D. Tyler, DVM, PhD, DACVP (Clinical and Anatomic
    Pathology), DABT**
Adjunct Professor
Department of Veterinary Pathobiology
Center for Veterinary Health Sciences
Oklahoma State University
Stillwater, Oklahoma
&
Tamil Nadu Veterinary and Animal Sciences University
Madras Veterinary College
Vepery, Chennai, India

Consulting Editor:
Dennis B. DeNicola, DVM, PhD, DACVP
Clinical Pathologist
Chief Veterinary Educator
IDEXX Laboratories, Inc.
Westbrook, Maine

ELSEVIER

3251 Riverport Lane
St. Louis, MO 63043

ATLAS OF CANINE AND FELINE PERIPHERAL BLOOD SMEARS
Edition 1

Notice

Knowledge and best practice in this field are constantly changing. As new research and
experience broaden our knowledge, changes in practice, treatment and drug therapy may
become necessary or appropriate. Readers are advised to check the most current information
provided (i) on procedures featured or (ii) by the manufacturer of each product to be
administered, to verify the recommended dose or formula, the method and duration of
administration, and contraindications. It is the responsibility of the practitioner, relying on their
own experience and knowledge of the patient, to make diagnoses, to determine dosages and the
best treatment for each individual patient, and to take all appropriate safety precautions. To the
fullest extent of the law, neither the Publisher nor the Editor assumes any liability for any injury
and/or damage to persons or property arising out of or related to any use of the material
contained in this book.

The Publisher

Library of Congress Cataloging-in-Publication Data

Valenciano, Amy C., author.
  Atlas of canine and feline peripheral blood smears / Amy C. Valenciano, Rick L. Cowell,
Theresa E. Rizzi, Ronald D. Tyler.
     p. ; cm.
  ISBN 978-0-323-04468-4 (alk. paper)
  I. Cowell, Rick L., author. II. Rizzi, Theresa E., author. III. Tyler, Ronald D., author. IV. Title.
  [DNLM: 1. Clinical Laboratory Techniques—Atlases. 2. Blood Cells—pathology—Atlases.
3. Blood Cells—ultrastructure—Atlases. 4. Cat Diseases—blood—Atlases. 5. Dog Diseases—
blood—Atlases. SF 772.67]
  SF769.5
  636.089'607561—dc23

                                                                                    2013012786

Vice President and Publisher: Linda Duncan
Content Strategy Director: Penny Rudolph
Content Development Specialist: Brandi Graham
Publishing Services Manager: Catherine Jackson
Project Manager: Sara Alsup
Designer: Jessica Williams

Printed in India

Last digit is the print number: 9 8 7 6

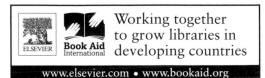

PREFACE

The Hematology Atlas of Canine and Feline Peripheral Blood Smears is created to be a "scopeside" visual atlas of normal and abnormal findings on dog and cat peripheral blood smears. Our aim is to provide veterinary students, veterinary technicians, practicing veterinarians, and veterinary residents with a large number of logically organized, high quality photomicrographs that are useful in learning to identify normal and abnormal peripheral blood findings and enjoyable to view. Each entity is fully characterized by multiple photomicrographs, taken at varying magnifications and encompassing variations in morphological features. Additionally, there are several special mosaic photomicrographs constructed of similar-appearing and often confused elements that enables careful comparison for quick microscopic differentiation. The concise text provides a quick and detailed description of each microscopic finding being emphasized to compliment the corresponding photomicrographs.

Emphasized are normal cellular findings and common abnormal findings, in particular, RBC and WBC morphology changes, hemoparasites, and infectious agents. A section on leukemia is provided to offer an overview of the different types of leukemias in dogs and cats, with an emphasis on the challenges of differentiating between the different cellular origins of leukemia based solely on light microscopy and thus the need for specialist review and further diagnostics. The authors sincerely hope this atlas will provide a means to develop a strong foundation in blood smear evaluation, and serve as valued reference for anyone interested in hematopathology.

ACKNOWLEDGMENTS

We thank our families for their support and understanding. Many other people deserve acknowledgement and sincere thanks also. These include Elsevier's excellent editors and staff, and the many veterinary pathologists at IDEXX laboratories and other colleagues who sent slides or pictures for use in the text, especially: Drs. Debbie Bernreuter, Dean Cornwell, Jim Mathews, Desire Lipscomb, Liz Little, Jennifer Neel, Natalie Courtman, Carrie Flint, Dennis DeNicola, Shanon Zablotsky, and Kari Velguth and Ms. Joan Shewmaker. We especially appreciate and recognize the editing work of Drs. Dave Fisher and Pat McManus who served as additional reviewers for this atlas.

Finally, we would like to thank IDEXX Laboratories for generously supporting veterinary education and this book in particular.

Amy C. Valenciano
Rick L. Cowell
Theresa E. Rizzi
Ronald D. Tyler

Supported in part by IDEXX Laboratories as part of their commitment to Veterinarians, Veterinary Technicians, and Veterinary Medical Education.

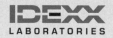

To Dr. Rick Cowell, an inspiration and excellent pathologist and mentor. Thank you for sharing your projects, insights, and laughter. It was an honor to work alongside you in creating this wonderful atlas. I dedicate my efforts to God and my family: Daniel (husband), Avery (daughter), Ty (son), Bonny (twin) and my dear parents. I thank my wonderful mentors especially Drs. Dave Fisher, Sonjia Shelly, Carol Grindem, Jan Andrews, Mary Jo Burkhard, Gregg Dean, Christine Stanton, and Lon Rich. I also thank IDEXX laboratories for supporting academic growth and for promoting excellence in veterinary pathology.

Amy Valenciano

To my parents who taught me the value of honesty
and instilled in me a work ethic that has served me well through the years.
To my wife (Annette) and daughter (Anne) who have continually given support,
meaning and inspiration to my life.
To my daughter (Rebecca) who showed me the face of true courage, and taught me to laugh and love even in the worst of times. While she lost her battle with cancer at the age of 11 her memories and life lessons will forever be remembered.
To the many outstanding veterinary clinical pathologists I have had the
opportunity to learn from especially, Drs. Ronald D. Tyler,
James Meinkoth, and Dennis DeNicola.
To the many veterinary practitioners, residents, and students who taught
me much more than I could ever have hoped to teach them, and have
become colleagues and friends.
To IDEXX Laboratories for their continued support of veterinary education and especially to Dr. Dean Cornwell for his support and encouragement.

Rick Cowell

To Deb, for your enduring love and support.
To my son, Aiden, who reminds me to laugh often and who always makes me proud.

Theresa E. Rizzi

To my mother who gave me my core tenants of faith, honesty and respect; my wonderful wife, Reba, for her patience and support; my children who have made my life truly wonderful, exciting, and worthwhile; and the many exceptional colleagues who have taught, inspired and guided me—especially Roger Panciera for his mentorship and Rick Cowell for his many contributions to my development as a person and pathologist and, most of all, his friendship through the years.

Ronald D. Tyler

CONTENTS

INTRODUCTION: BLOOD SMEAR PREPARATION AND EXAMINATION

Overview

Evaluation of blood smears is a fundamental step in overall health assessment and is included in standard hematologic profiles and as part of the diagnostic evaluation of virtually every ill patient. In addition to being a means of obtaining the differential white blood cell (WBC) count (i.e., determination of the distribution of the different types of leukocytes, both as percentages and counts per microliter [μL]), blood smear examination may yield a broad range of diagnostic information. For example, altered red blood cell (RBC) morphology may suggest chronic blood loss, exposure to endogenous and exogenous toxins, disorders of vasculature, or immune-mediated hemolysis. Changes in WBC morphology may be the earliest laboratory finding of inflammation and may be diagnostic for certain inherited conditions and leukemias. Some changes occur in leukocyte maturity, morphology, and type that may only be detected through microscopic evaluation of peripheral blood smears (i.e., neutrophilic left-shift, neutrophilic toxic change, and the presence of circulating mast cells). In some cases, infectious agents, pathognomonic cellular inclusions, and neoplastic cells are observed on blood films, yielding an immediate, definitive diagnosis. In addition, monitoring changes found in peripheral blood may help determine a patient's treatment, response to therapy, and short-term and long-term prognoses.

Blood smear evaluation should be performed as part of every complete blood count (CBC), either in-house or in an outside laboratory. Evaluation provides morphologic confirmation of hematologic parameters, assurance of the quality of values obtained from automated analyzers, and additional important information not given by automated methods. The value of blood smear review is maximized when the information is correlated with the patient's medical history, current and previous laboratory findings, and physical examination findings.

Blood smear preparation is easy and inexpensive, and experience in evaluation is readily acquired with adequate background information and regular practice. This introduction describes applicable techniques and interpretations of canine and feline blood smears. A brief introduction to the integration of findings from blood smear evaluations with other values in the CBC is included.

Equipment and Supplies

An essential piece of equipment for blood smear evaluation is a well-maintained, binocular microscope with high-quality 10, 20, 40 or 50 (ideally, oil-immersion 50×), and 100× (oil-immersion) objectives. Additionally, clean glass slides and good-quality, fresh stains and Coplin jars are needed for in-house staining.

Standard plain or frosted glass slides may be used directly from the package without special treatment or cleaning. Slides with frosted ends facilitate labeling with patient information. Slide surfaces should be free of dust, fingerprints, and residue from detergent, alcohol, or tap water. The use of special cytologic adhesives may result in background staining and are not recommended. An ample supply of slides facilitates preparation of multiple smears per sample, avoiding the frustration of interpreting any poorly made smears. These additional smears may also be reserved for alternative types of staining or, if indicated, a specialist's review.

Sample Collection

Ideally, blood samples should be collected on the first attempt from a medium to large vein of a calm patient. Ethylenediaminetetraacetic acid (EDTA) is the preferred anticoagulant for blood used in cytologic preparations. The liquid form of EDTA disperses more rapidly in samples and may be preferable to the powder form, particularly for feline blood, but both forms of EDTA preserve general cellular morphology in refrigerated samples for up to 4 hours. In either case, adequate mixing is essential and is accomplished by gently inverting the tube 6 to 10 times. Alternatively, blood without an anticoagulant may be placed directly from the collection needle onto the slide. This is preferred by some because of possible morphologic alterations caused by the EDTA and is particularly useful if sample volume is limited. Samples collected from superficial skin-puncture wounds, clipped toenails (due to excessive contamination with tissue procoagulants), and blood anticoagulated with heparin (a relatively poor preservative of cellular morphology and staining characteristics) are less acceptable. Blood anticoagulated with citrate may be used to evaluate cell morphology on blood smears; however, the required 10% sample dilution interferes with cell count estimates.

Collection of blood in proper proportion to anticoagulant is facilitated by the use of commercial vacutainers. This is essential to avoid certain artifacts of cell morphology and also to achieve accurate cell counts, which may be affected by overfilling and underfilling the tube.

Smear Preparation

The goal of blood smear preparation is to spread the cells (RBC, WBC, and platelets), so a large, uniform, single layer (monolayer) of cells is created. In the monolayer, RBC should be side by side, yet infrequently touching, and should be devoid of large spaces without cells. In the monolayer, WBCs flatten and stain well, allowing good evaluation of cytoplasmic and nuclear detail. WBCs will be evenly distributed, allowing accurate differential counts to be performed and promoting examination of WBC, RBC, and platelet morphologies. Inclusions such as rickettsial and viral inclusions may be readily identified. In thick areas of the smear, cells often are too contracted, distorted, and poorly stained for reliable evaluation. In excessively thin areas of the smear and in the feathered edge, cells are often distorted, damaged, and ruptured, prohibiting reliable classification and morphologic evaluation. Also, a differential WBC count performed near or in the feathered edge results in skewing toward the larger cell types.

Well-made smears are essential for reliable identification, quantification, and evaluation of peripheral blood cells. Smears may be prepared on glass slides or coverslips. The glass slide technique is generally easier and more reliable than preparing smears on coverslips. Glass slides may also be processed through automatic stainers and are most suitable for laboratories using such equipment. However, the coverslip method generally results in more uniform WBC distribution and less trauma to fragile blood components such as large or neoplastic cells. For both methods, blood samples should be fresh and adequately mixed just prior to smear preparation, and smears should be completely air-dried before staining.

The blood smear preparation technique should be learned well, as it is necessary for reliable in-house blood smear examination and hemogram results from samples submitted to referral laboratories. At least one freshly prepared (in-house) blood smear should accompany all EDTA-anticoagulated blood samples submitted to referral laboratories for CBC. Failure to submit a premade blood smear may result in several artifacts; for example, blood parasites (e.g., *Mycoplasma hemofelis*) may fall off the RBC surfaces, resulting in false-negative results; platelet numbers will decrease and may cause platelet estimates to be falsely decreased; and WBCs become pyknotic (secondary to aging), and when 10% or more of the WBCs are pyknotic, the differential count is invalid.

Smears are prepared on glass slides by placing a drop of blood (2 to 3 mm in diameter) on the broad face of the slide about 1 to 1.5 cm from the frosted border (or edge of a nonfrosted slide). Another clean, dry slide (spreader slide) is held loosely against the surface of the first slide at a 30-degree angle and drawn smoothly toward the blood drop. The spreader slide should be brought to a position where it just meets, but is not drawn into, the blood drop. When the spreader slide makes contact with the blood, capillary action immediately distributes the blood between the two slides. Then, with no downward pressure, the spreader slide is quickly and smoothly swept across the remaining length of the underlying slide.

Ideally, blood smears have a smooth transition from the thick region to the feathered edge and cover an area one half the length and slightly less than the width of the slide. If the edge of the blood film is blunt instead of feathered, the second slide was probably raised off the first before the blood was spread completely. Unequal smear thickness usually results from the spreader slide being held at too obtuse an angle or placing too much pressure on the first slide while spreading the blood. Too much pressure on the second slide may also result in WBCs clumping along the smear's feathered edge. Too little pressure may result in short, thick smears. Smear thickness may also be affected by the viscosity of the blood sample. Adjusting the angle at which the second slide is held against the first may help compensate for very viscous (hemoconcentrated) or thin (anemic) blood samples. A more obtuse (40- to 45-degree) angle between the two slides makes thicker smears for very anemic blood, and an angle less than 30 degrees may be necessary for preparing smears of severely hemoconcentrated blood. Smears need to be thoroughly air-dried before staining; those that are thick may require additional drying time (and additional time in fixative and stain).

Common problems in blood smear technique include unclean slides, placing too large a drop of blood on the blood smear slide, pulling the prep slide too far back, excessive pressure, slow movement of the prep slide forward, and jerky or uneven forward movement of the prep slide.

Unclean microscope slides may cause spaces devoid of cells to be scattered throughout the smear, prohibit smooth movement of the prep slide, and impair the staining of portions or the entire smear.

Using a drop of blood that is too large causes the smear to be too thick and to extend too far down the blood smear slide. Often, the blood smear extends to the end of the slide without formation of a monolayer, precluding reliable microscopic examination.

Pulling the prep slide too far back causes blood to flow underneath the prep slide. When the prep slide is moved forward, plasma and smaller cells (i.e., platelets, erythrocytes, and small lymphocytes) pass back under the prep slide more easily than do larger cells (i.e., neutrophils and monocytes). As a result, WBCs are unevenly distributed with small lymphocytes being in excess in the earlier formed portion of the smear and neutrophils and monocytes being in excess in the later formed portion of the smear (i.e., feathered edge). Obviously, these smears may give misleading differential WBC counts.

Excessive pressure on the prep slide causes uneven WBC spreading, where most of the WBCs become concentrated at the feathered edge. Also, with extreme pressure it may be difficult to rapidly and smoothly move the prep slide forward. Thus, excessive pressure may lead to irregular smears and uneven distribution of WBC types, resulting in inaccurate differential WBC counts.

Stains

As with cytologic preparations, Romanowsky-type stains (Wright; Wright-Giemsa) are good general stains for microscopic blood smear evaluation. Quick Romanowsky-type stains (Diff-Quik) are advantageous because they are less sensitive to solution pH and staining time and less susceptible to precipitate formation compared with Wright stains. However, most quick stains are also less effective at demonstrating polychromasia of immature erythrocytes, granules in some cells (i.e., granular lymphocytes and mast cells), and toxic change in neutrophils. Thus, whenever possible, Wright stains are preferred.

Different brands of Wright and Wright-Giemsa stains are available, and following the manufacturer's staining protocol for each type is advised. In general, staining is achieved by first dipping the air-dried slides into a methanol-containing Coplin jar for fixation (approximately 30 seconds). After fixation, the slides are dipped into Coplin jars containing the stain reagent. Some manufacturers have one type of stain reagent, others have two. After staining, the slides are dipped into Coplin jars containing buffer and then rinsed with water (tap, deionized, or a combination of tap and deionized water). The slides may be dried by blotting with bibulous paper or placed upright on an absorptive surface to hasten drying. A blow dryer set on low power and held 8 to 10 inches from the slide also shortens drying time.

Quick stain methods vary somewhat and should be used according to manufacturer's recommendations. Diff-Quik requires three separate solutions: (1) an alcohol fixative, (2) a methylene blue dye mixture, and (3) an eosin-containing solution. The smear is slowly dipped and slightly swished five or more times into each solution in sequence, with one edge of the slide briefly blotted between solutions. For each step, the fluid should drain smoothly off the slide between dips, with no bubbling or unevenness, before proceeding to the next solution. Tap or distilled water is used to rinse the slide after the last solution and before air-drying.

Hematologic Reference Intervals

Reference intervals, which are found in publications and texts, provided by a reference laboratory, or provided by manufacturers of bench-top analyzers, are generally reliable. Certain physiologic factors occasionally cause a healthy patient's hematologic values to deviate from reference intervals. For example, very young animals are rapidly expanding their vascular space and tend to have relatively low hematocrits. Young animals are also actively replacing fetal RBCs with adult RBCs and also have greater erythrocytic anisocytosis and polychromasia and a higher frequency of nucleated RBCs compared with mature animals. Relatively high lymphocyte counts are also common in young animals, and lymphopenia is suggested in puppies and kittens less than 6 months of age if lymphocyte counts drop below 2000 cells/μL. Transient elevations above the reference interval for lymphocyte counts are common in excited or vigorously exercised patients, especially if they are immature. This epinephrine-induced response may also result in temporarily increased counts of other WBC types in the peripheral blood of healthy patients. At least one canine breed, the Greyhound (and potentially other sight hounds as well), has hematologic reference intervals reported to fall slightly outside of reference intervals commonly used for the species. Although these normal physiologic conditions should be considered, they generally explain less than 5% of the patient values that fall outside reference intervals for any single hematologic result.

SECTION 1:
GENERAL ASSESSMENT

Blood Smears

DISTINCTIVE FEATURES: Blood smears have three major areas: (1) the thick inner area (body); (2) the monolayer; and (3) the feathered edge (the most external area). The inner area is the thickest area of the smear, and cells are usually too contracted, distorted, or poorly stained for reliable evaluation. The monolayer is the best area for cell morphology evaluation and differential cell counts, whereas the feathered edge is the best area to search for organisms (i.e., microfilaria), clumped platelets, and large atypical cells, neoplastic cells, or both. Blood smears should have a smooth transition in thickness from the proximal end to the distal end of the smear and have an adequate monolayer for evaluation of cell distribution and morphology. The monolayer is found within the distal half of the smear adjacent to the feathered edge and is luminescent when the unstained slide is held under indirect light.

DIAGNOSTIC SIGNIFICANCE: Initially, the entire smear should be quickly scanned using the 10 or 20× objective from the thickest region to the feathered edge. At this low magnification, blood films may be checked for staining, overall thickness, smooth transitions in thickness, cell distribution, adequacy of the monolayer area, and general appearance of the background. The feathered edge may be scanned at low power for platelet clumps, large parasites and large, atypical nucleated cells.

A patient's hematocrit may be crudely estimated by examining a blood smear at low magnification. This estimate assumes that smear thickness was not increased or decreased to compensate for anemia or hemoconcentration by increasing or decreasing the angle of the spreader slide. Blood films from nonanemic animals generally have red blood cells (RBCs) that are closely apposed in the monolayer as well as several RBC layers at the thick end of the smear that obstruct penetrance of most of the condenser light. In contrast, smears from animals that are moderately to markedly anemic usually have RBCs that are widely separated from one another in the monolayer and only one to two RBC layers in the thick end of the smear that allow considerable condenser light to penetrate. In smears prepared from hemoconcentrated specimens, the monolayer will occupy a relatively smaller zone and cells may be crowded and difficult to evaluate. Estimates should ultimately be checked against the patient's measured hematocrit or packed cell volume (PCV).

Monolayer

DISTINCTIVE FEATURES: In the monolayer, blood cells are present in a single layer. Cells should be side by side, but infrequently touching, and should not be distorted. Also, the monolayer should be devoid of large spaces without cells.

DIAGNOSTIC SIGNIFICANCE: The monolayer represents the limited region where cell morphology is most reliably evaluated. White blood cells (WBCs) should be fairly uniformly distributed within this region. WBC estimates, differential platelet estimates, and examination of WBC, RBC, and platelet morphologies should be done in the monolayer. In the monolayer, WBCs flatten and stain well, allowing good evaluation of cytoplasmic and nuclear detail. Also, inclusions such as rickettsial and viral inclusions may be readily identified.

On a well-made blood smear, the total WBC and differential cell counts may be estimated or simply classified as low, normal, or high by examining the monolayer of the smear using the 40× or 50× objective, whereas platelet frequency is best estimated using the 100× objective.

Plate 1-1   Normal Monolayer

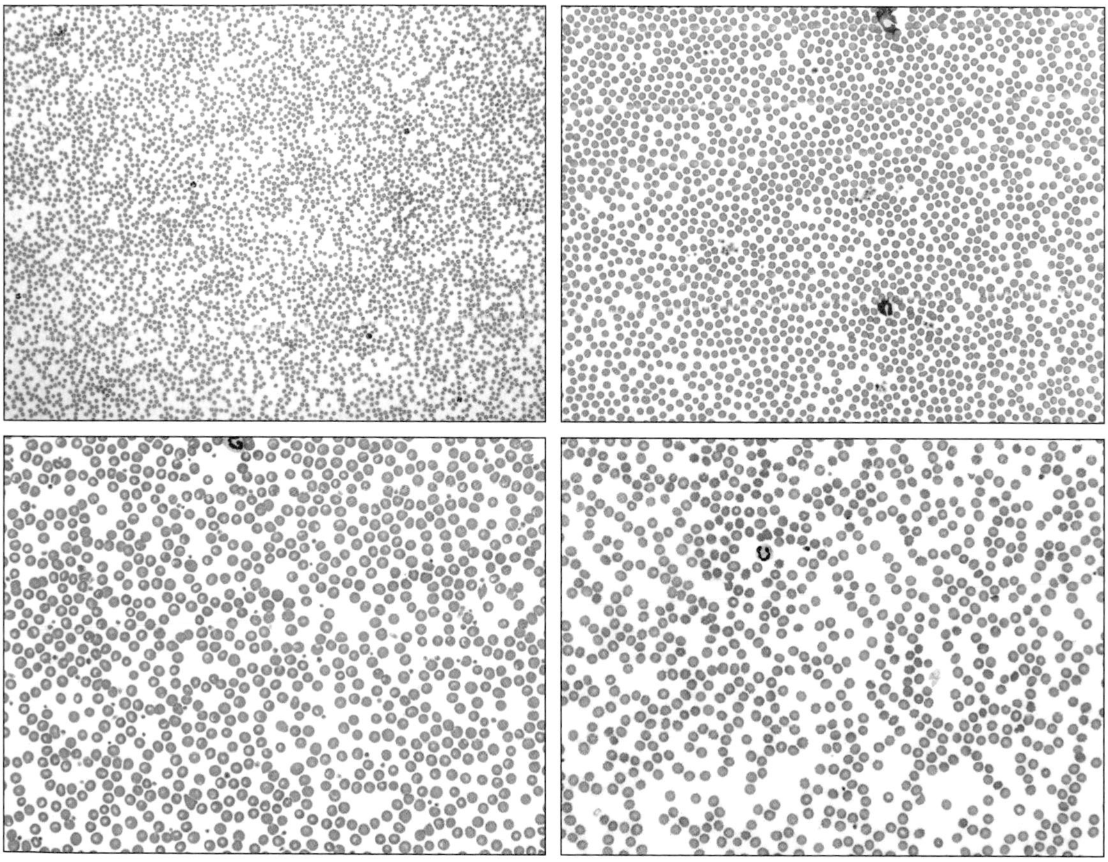

Plate 1-1 Normal Monolayer *(con't)*

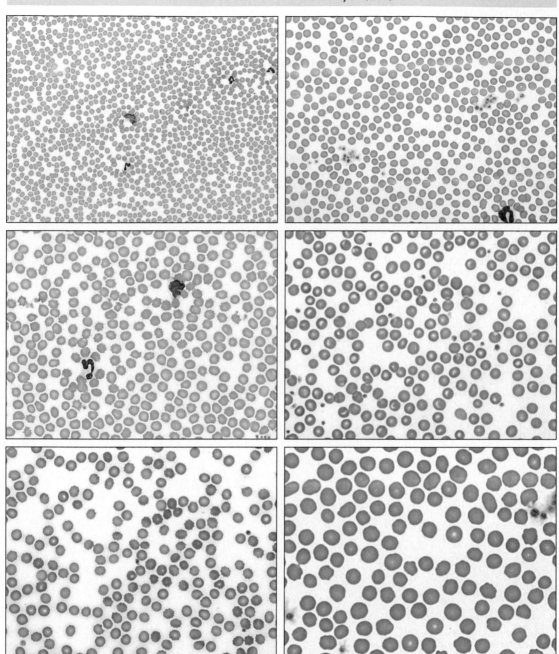

Feathered Edge

DISTINCTIVE FEATURES: The feathered edge is the gently tapered end of the smear, located opposite the point of application of the blood drop.

DIAGNOSTIC SIGNIFICANCE: Large structures such as platelet clumps, microfilaria, cells containing infectious agents, and large, normal or neoplastic nucleated cells may be concentrated in this area. Thus, microscopic examination of the feathered edge is essential.

If large platelet clumps are found at the feathered edge, this may account for a low or low-normal platelet estimate in the monolayer when evaluating platelet numbers and may also indicate that an instrument-generated platelet count may not be valid. Large neoplastic nucleated cells may be found in low or high numbers in this area, suggesting leukemia or circulating neoplastic cells from nonhematopoietic neoplasia (i.e., mast cell tumor and lymphoma). Large parasites, in particular, microfilaria, may be located in this region as well. Cells with intracellular organisms such as leukocytes containing *Histoplasma* organisms and RBCs containing *Babesia* spp. hemoparasites may concentrate in the feathered edge. A differential WBC count may be inaccurately skewed toward larger cell types if the differential is performed mostly at the feathered edge. Also, in the feathered edge, cells are often distorted, damaged, or ruptured, prohibiting reliable classification and morphologic evaluation.

If excessive pressure is applied to the spreader smear during smear preparation, most of the nucleated cells will end up in the feathered edge of the smear. Estimates of the total WBC count and determination of percentages of the different types of leukocytes based only on examination of the monolayer of the smear will be inaccurate. A total WBC count may be attempted by evaluating the number of nucleated cells in the feathered edge and monolayer of the smear at 10× magnification.

Plate 1-2   Normal Feathered Edge

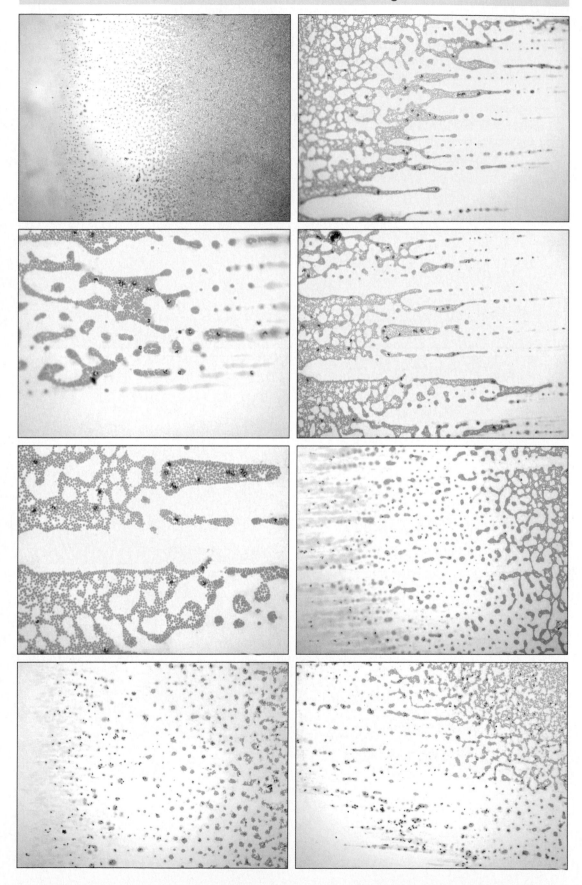

Body

DISTINCTIVE FEATURES: The body is the thick inner part of the smear. The cells are touching, and no space exists between cells.

DIAGNOSTIC SIGNIFICANCE: The cells in the body of the smear are distorted and compressed, prohibiting evaluation of cell morphology and performing a differential WBC count. Sometimes, large parasites such as microfilaria may be found in this region on a low-power scan.

Plate 1-3 Normal Body

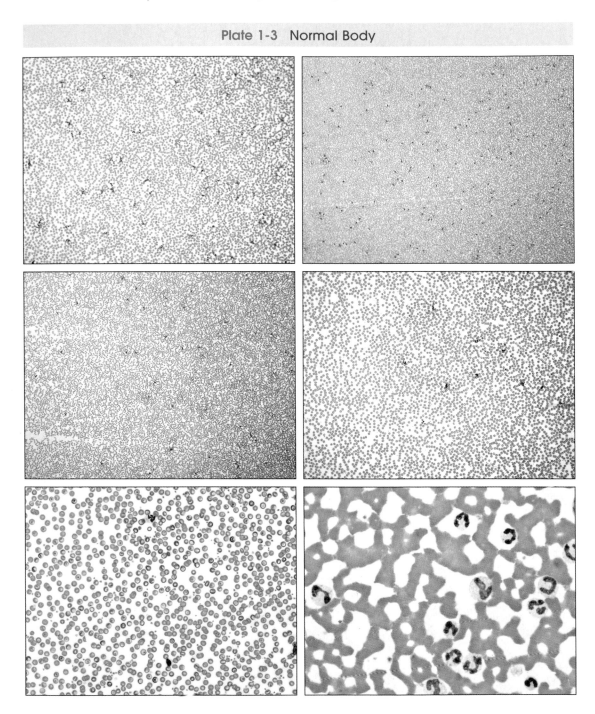

Plate 1-3 Normal Body *(con't)*

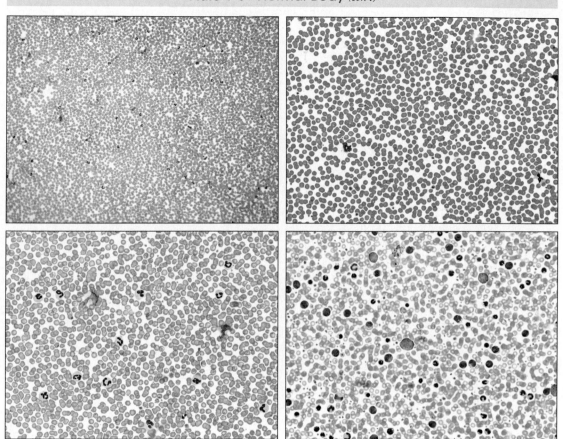

Background

DISTINCTIVE FEATURES: The background of the smear should be colorless and free of stain debris or precipitant.

Increased Basophilia

DISTINCTIVE FEATURES: The background of the smear stains a basophilic hue.

DIAGNOSTIC SIGNIFICANCE: If the background of the smear stains more intensely than normal, increased plasma protein concentration should be considered, warranting evaluation for hyperglobulinemia.

Plate 1-4 Increased Background Basophilia

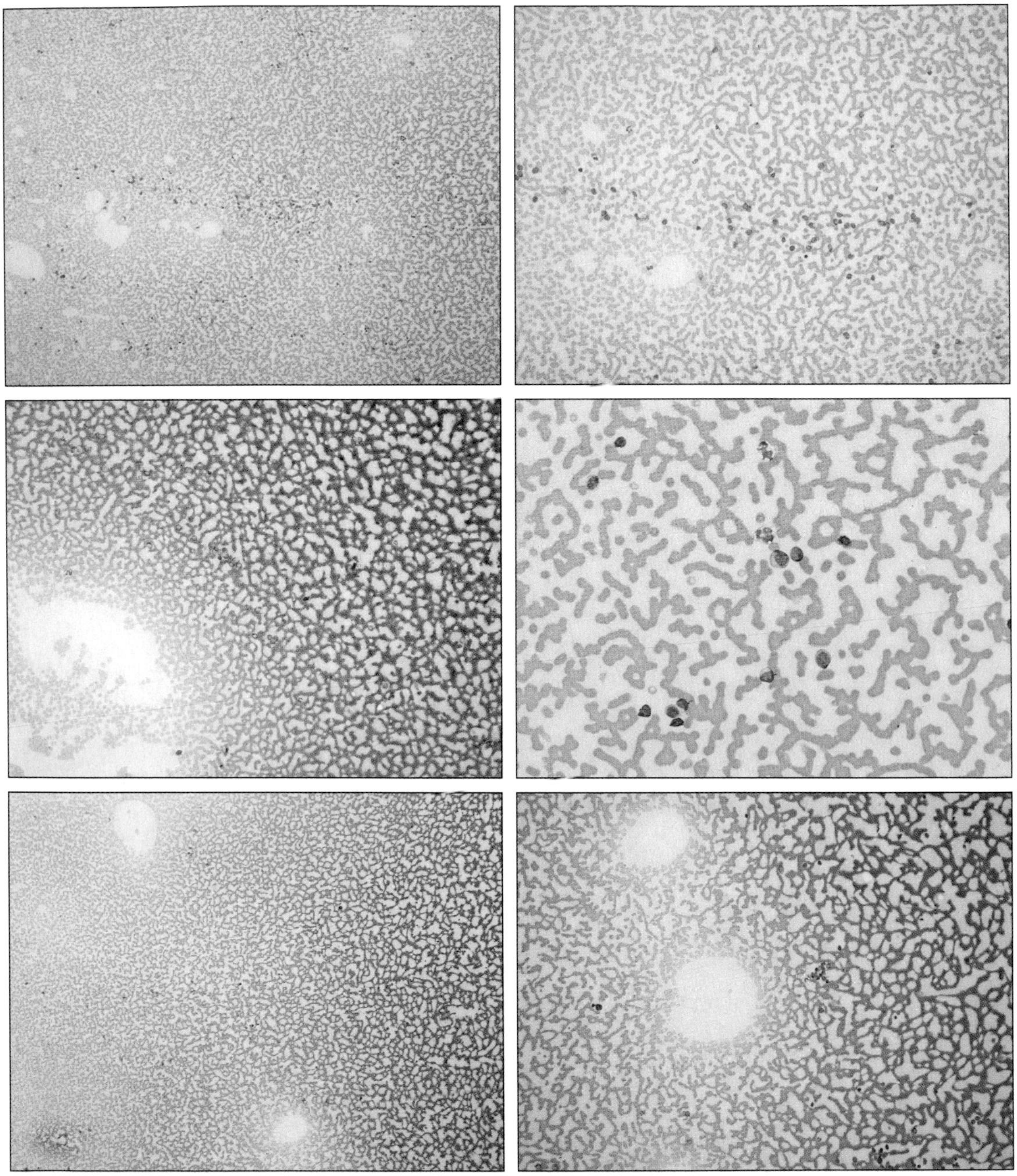

Plate 1-4 Increased Background Basophilia *(con't)*

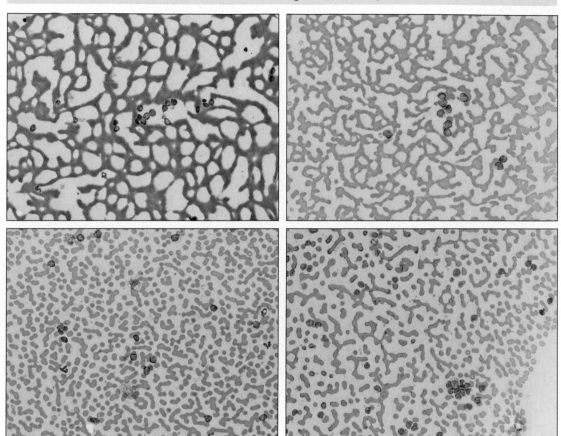

Cytoplasmic Fragments

DISTINCTIVE FEATURES: With some acute leukemias, the background may contain cytoplasmic fragments (sometimes called *lymphoglandular bodies*) formed from rapidly dividing or ruptured neoplastic cells.

DIAGNOSTIC SIGNIFICANCE: These are characterized by small, basophilic, anucleate blebs that could be mistaken for platelets. If cytoplasmic fragments are found, assess the slide carefully for circulating neoplastic cells.

Plate 1-5 Cytoplasmic Fragments

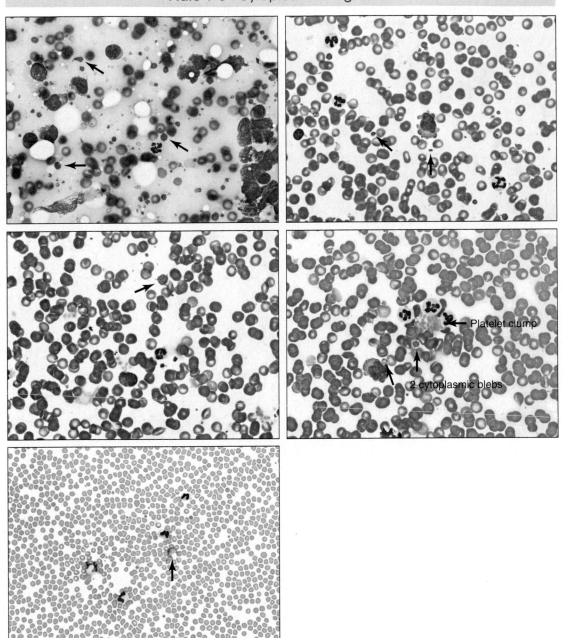

Infectious Agents

DISTINCTIVE FEATURES: Free hemoparasites may be found in the background, warranting careful microscopic assessment of the extracellular space. Section VI, Extracellular Organisms, contains detailed information on the different types of infectious agents that may be found free in the background of blood films.

Plate 1-6 Extracellular Infectious Agents
A, Microfilaria **B,** Trypanosomes **C,** Spirochetes **D,** Bacteria

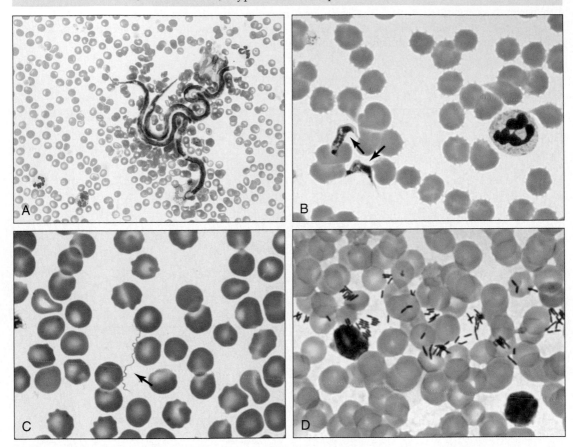

Stain Precipitation

DISTINCTIVE FEATURES: Stain precipitant is usually dark blue, fine, and found in small clusters.

DIAGNOSTIC SIGNIFICANCE: Stain precipitant may be confused with external parasites (especially *Myco-plasma hemofelis* organisms that have dislodged from the RBC surface), and when overlapping or adjacent to RBCs, the stain may be confused with hemoparasites.

Plate 1-7   Stain Precipitant

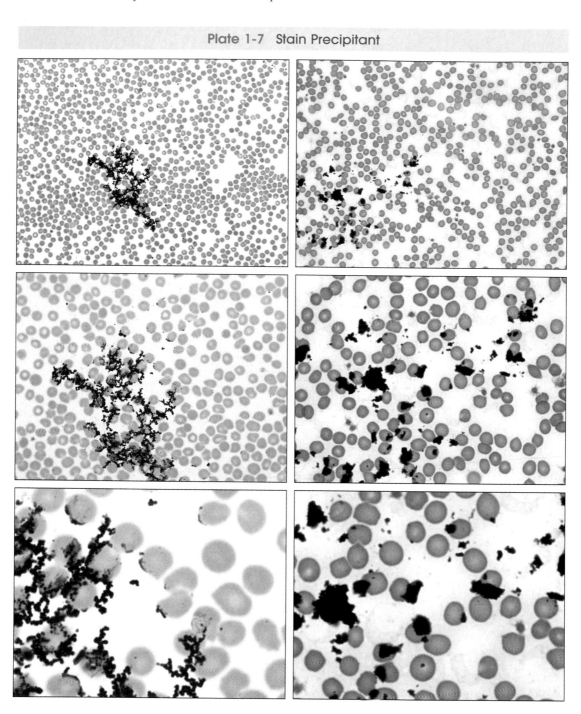

Plate 1-7 Stain Precipitant *(con't)*

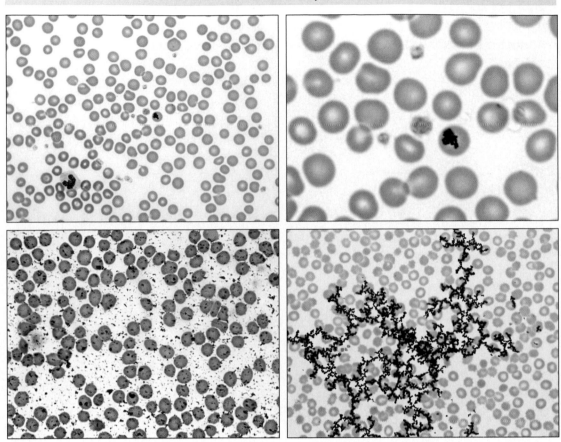

Make sure not to confuse stain precipitate with **A,** *Mycoplasma hemocanis*; **B,** *Mycoplasma hemofelis*; **C,** Extracellular bacteria.

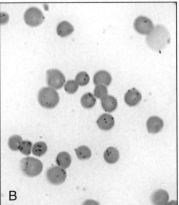
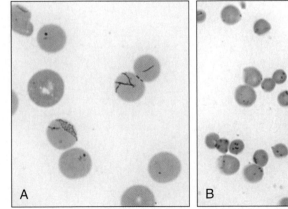
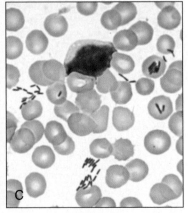

Fibrin

DISTINCTIVE FEATURES: Fibrin may be found on the feathered edge of the smear, sometimes with entangled platelets. Fibrin forms large, slender, homogeneous, pale blue, intertwining strands.

DIAGNOSTIC SIGNIFICANCE: Fibrin should not be confused with microfilaria.

Plate 1-8 Fibrin

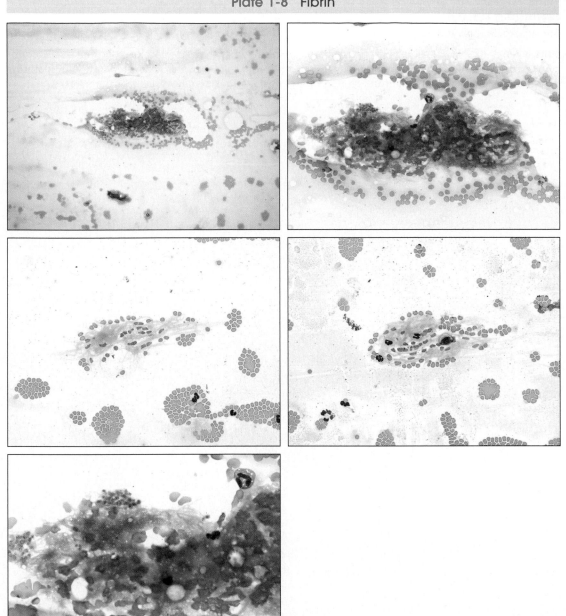

Skin Contaminants

DISTINCTIVE FEATURES: Skin contaminants are individualized, polygonal to flattened, basophilic, anucleate superficial squamous epithelial cells.

DIAGNOSTIC SIGNIFICANCE: Skin contaminants are from either the patient's skin obtained during venipuncture or, more frequently, from fingerprints made on the slide during slide preparation or staining. These are external contaminants and should not be mistaken for neoplastic cells or parasites.

Plate 1-9 Skin Contaminants

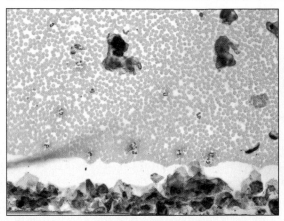 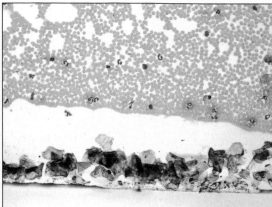

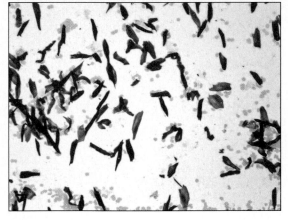

SECTION 2:
RED BLOOD CELLS

Normal Morphology (Discocytes and Normocytes)

DISTINCTIVE FEATURES: Mature canine and feline erythrocytes are anucleate, red, disc-like cells (discocytes). Canine red blood cells (RBCs) are approximately 7 micrometers (µm) in diameter and shaped like biconcave discs with prominent central pallor. Feline erythrocytes are smaller, approximately 6 µm in diameter, and more "cup" shaped, so they lack the prominent central pallor seen in canine RBCs.

DIAGNOSTIC SIGNIFICANCE: Discocytes are the expected finding in healthy nonanemic dogs and cats but can be the predominant RBC morphology observed in many disease states as well.

Plate 2-1
A, Canine red blood cell (RBC) **B,** Normal feline RBC

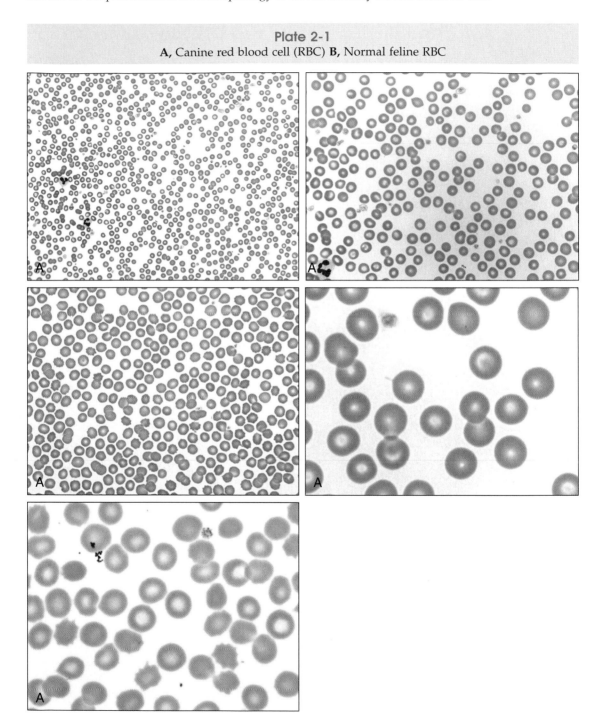

Plate 2-1
A, Canine red blood cell (RBC) **B,** Normal feline RBC *(con't)*

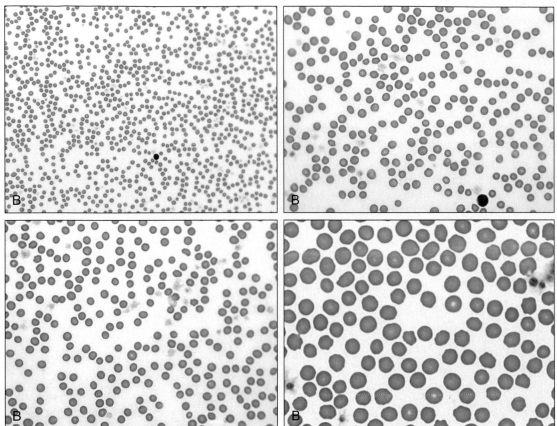

Anemia

DISTINCTIVE FEATURES: Anemia is a decrease in numbers of RBCs compared with established reference intervals and can be estimated by blood smear evaluation or quantitated by RBC count, hemoglobin concentration, and measurement of the hematocrit.

DIAGNOSTIC SIGNIFICANCE: Two general mechanisms of anemia, each with several etiologies, exist. The first mechanism is decreased RBC production from bone marrow failure or disease. Differentials could include immune-mediated mechanisms, toxins, drug effects, infectious agents (feline leukemia virus [FeLV], *Ehrlichia* spp.), endocrine disease, chronic liver and renal disease, and neoplasia (primary bone marrow neoplasia or metastatic neoplasia). The second major mechanism of anemia is increased RBC loss, which could be secondary to immune-mediated RBC destruction, hemolysis (viral, bacterial, or ehrlichial infections; RBC fragmentation; oxidative RBC damage), and acute and chronic blood loss (coagulopathies, trauma, blood sucking endoparasites and ectoparasites).

NEXT STEPS: When anemia is diagnosed, careful blood smear assessment of RBC morphology and investigation for hemoparasites are important for classifying the anemia and identifying the cause and to assess for evidence of RBC regeneration. Additionally, evaluation of platelet numbers and morphology and the white blood cell (WBC) line may help identify important etiologies of anemia.

Plate 2-2   Anemic Blood Smears

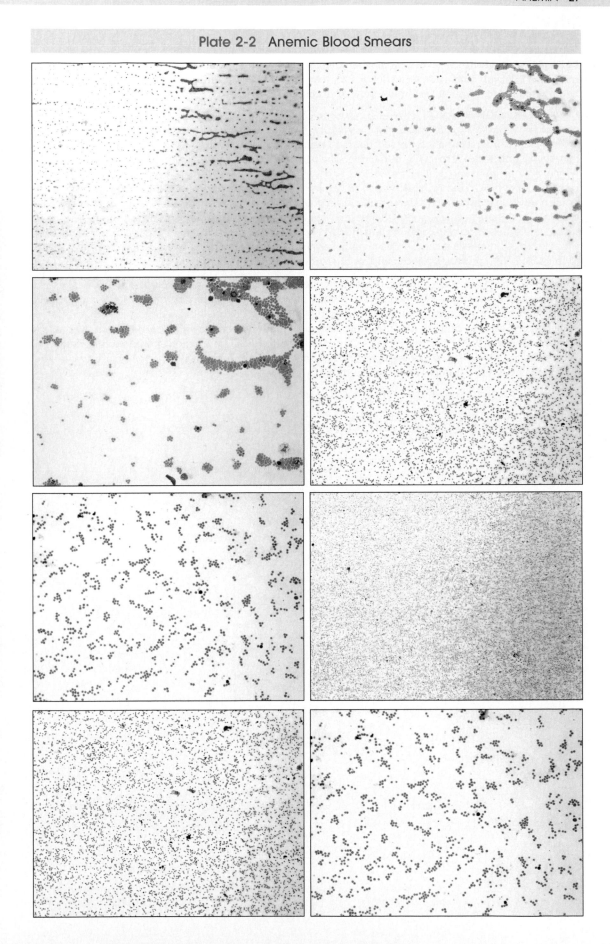

Polycythemia

DISTINCTIVE FEATURES: Polycythemia is an increase in the number of RBCs compared with established reference intervals and may be estimated by blood smear evaluation or quantitated by RBC count, hemoglobin concentration, and measurement of the hematocrit.

DIAGNOSTIC SIGNIFICANCE: The most common cause of polycythemia in dogs and cats is hemoconcentration secondary to decreased plasma volume (dehydration and endotoxic shock). A mild or moderate transient polycythemia may be secondary to epinephrine release (from excitement or fright), resulting in splenic contraction, especially in the dog. The last major category is from increased RBC production, which may be physiologically appropriate and inappropriate. Appropriate erythroid production is in response to hypoxia primarily secondary to cardiac disease, pulmonary disease, or both. Animals living at high altitudes and some canine breeds (Greyhound and other sight breeds) also have greater hematocrit values. Inappropriate polycythemia may result from inappropriate production of erythropoietin (responsible for stimulating RBC production in the marrow), as from renal cysts or tumors and some other types of neoplasia. Lastly, polycythemia vera (primary bone marrow neoplasia or leukemia) results in increased RBC production independent of erythropoietin.

NEXT STEPS: When polycythemia is identified, dehydration must first be excluded by physical examination and by checking blood chemistry parameters (total protein concentration, blood urea nitrogen [BUN]) and a urinalysis (urine specific gravity). If polycythemia is not secondary to dehydration, is persistent, and the patient does not live at high altitudes and is not a sight hound breed, then assessment for appropriate or inappropriate causes of increased RBC production should be considered and may include blood smear assessment, measurement of erythropoietin levels, bone marrow cytology, and exclusion of cardiac, pulmonary, and renal diseases.

Plate 2-3 Polycythemia

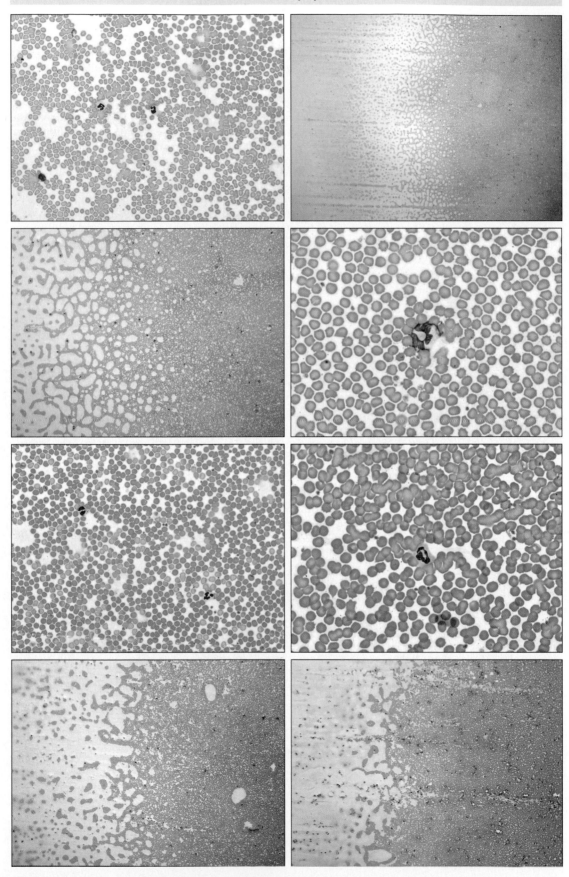

Morphologic Changes Associated with Disease

Rouleaux

DISTINCTIVE FEATURES: Groups of RBCs forming peculiar linear stacks in a conformation similar to a roll of coins, is called *rouleaux* and is secondary to the electrostatic association of RBCs. Rouleaux may be seen in the thick area of the smear in healthy cats but should not be present in the monolayer of the smear.

DIAGNOSTIC SIGNIFICANCE: Rouleaux may be seen occasionally in healthy dogs and especially cats. Increased rouleaux formation is occasionally observed in sick or debilitated dogs and cats with increased fibrinogen or globulin concentration. Rouleaux is generally associated with inflammatory conditions but also in some noninflammatory conditions such as lymphoproliferative disorders resulting in increased globulin production. Lipemic blood samples may cause increased rouleaux as well.

NEXT STEPS: Careful attention should be made to not confuse rouleaux with RBC agglutination. Rouleaux are orderly linear stacks of RBCs, whereas RBC agglutination is formed by grapelike RBC aggregates. To aid in differentiating between rouleaux and agglutination, a saline dilution test is useful. Rouleaux may be easily dissociated by dilution of RBCs in saline, whereas true agglutination persists despite saline dilution (for method, see Appendix). If rouleaux is confirmed, determine plasma or serum total protein, albumin, globulin, fibrinogen values and lipemic index, and investigate potential causes of any abnormalities found.

Plate 2-4 Rouleaux

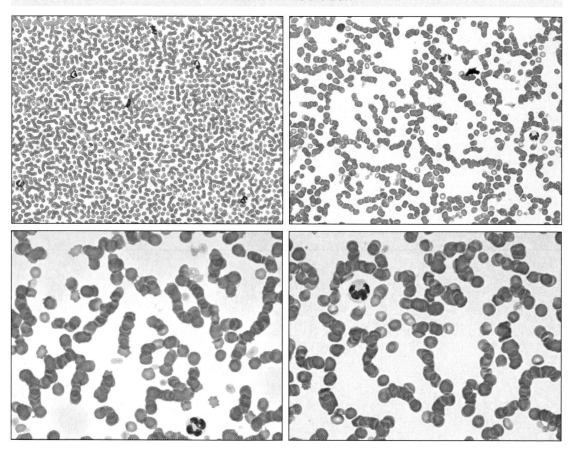

Plate 2-4   Rouleaux *(con't)*

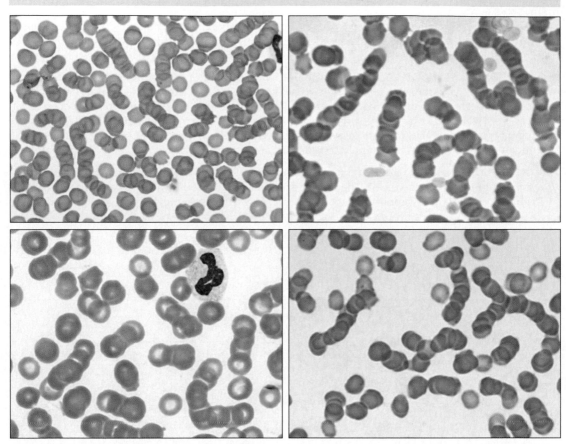

Make sure not to confuse rouleaux and agglutination.
A, Rouleaux **B,** Agglutination

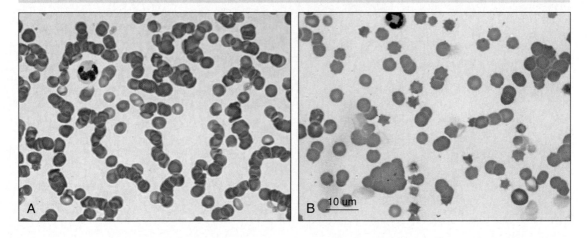

Agglutination

DISTINCTIVE FEATURES: Agglutination is a random, disorganized clumping of RBCs as opposed to the organized stack-of-coins formation seen with rouleaux formation. Agglutination is most prominent in the body of the blood film (thick area) and may occur in this area as an artifact. Agglutination is significant if found in the monolayer.

DIAGNOSTIC SIGNIFICANCE: Agglutination occurs when antibodies on one RBC bind to antigen on other RBCs, forming globular to amorphous, grapelike aggregates of RBCs. When present, RBC agglutination is supportive of immune-mediated hemolytic anemia (IMHA). Agglutination is not observed in most cases of IMHA, but when present, it occurs most commonly with immunoglobulin M (IgM) because of its pentavalent nature. However, extremely heavy IgG antibody coating of RBC membranes may cause agglutination. Agglutination is generally considered diagnostic of IMHA.

> **NEXT STEPS:** If necessary, agglutination may be differentiated from rouleaux formation by performing a saline dilution (dispersion) test. The presence of RBC agglutination warrants careful assessment of the blood film for other supportive evidence of IMHA such as spherocytes, and also for underlying causes of IMHA such as neoplastic cells and hemoparasites.

Plate 2-5   RBC Agglutination

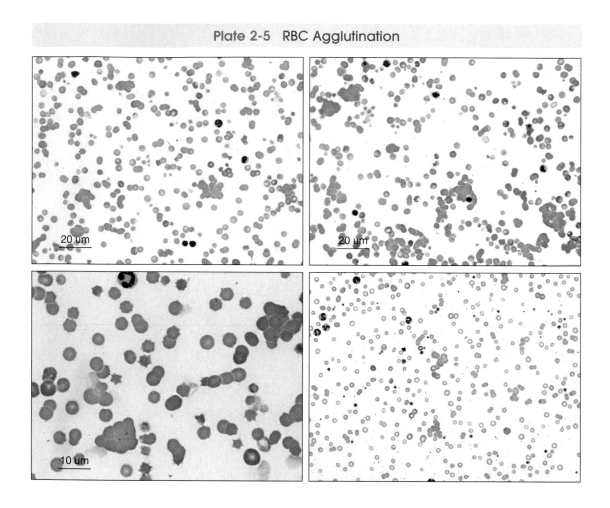

20 um

20 um

10 um

Plate 2-5   RBC Agglutination *(con't)*

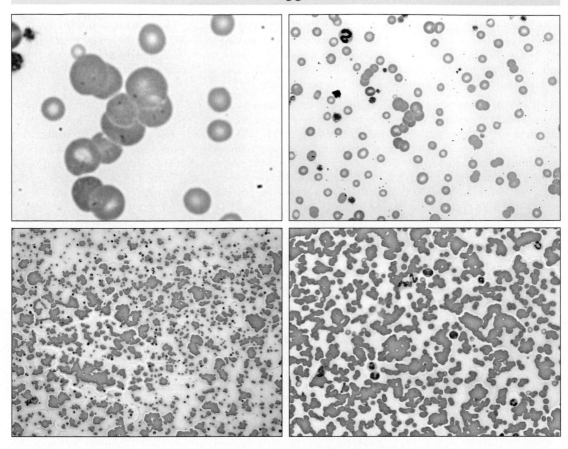

Make sure not to confuse agglutination with rouleaux.
A, Rouleaux **B,** Agglutination

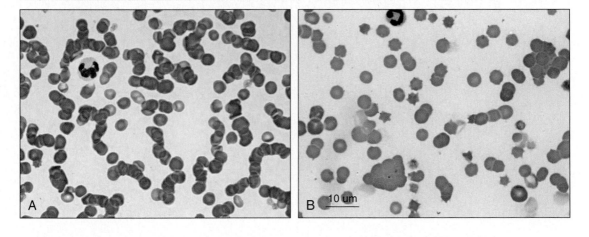

Polychromasia

DISTINCTIVE FEATURES: Polychromatophils are young, anucleate erythrocytes that stain both blue and pink (hence polychromatophilic), making the cell appear gray or bluish-red with Romanowsky-type stains. The blue color is caused by the presence of basophilic staining cellular organelles (ribosomes) that are broken down within 12 to 24 hours after release from bone marrow. Typically, polychromatophilic cells are larger than normochromic erythrocytes. Polychromatophil cells are counted as reticulocytes when stained with new methylene blue (see next section).

DIAGNOSTIC SIGNIFICANCE: Significant polychromasia indicates a regenerative bone marrow response to anemia. Hemorrhage and hemolysis are the two main causes of regenerative anemia and increased numbers of polychromatophilic RBCs. Remember that polychromasia does not occur instantly after hemorrhage or hemolysis but takes 2 to 4 days to increase the number of polychromatophilic erythrocytes in peripheral blood and may not exceed the reference interval or achieve maximum values for 5 to 7 days. Therefore, early or acute hemorrhagic or hemolytic anemias may have minimal polychromasia. Also, polychromatophilic RBCs are often difficult to differentiate from normochromic RBCs when smears are stained with rapid stains (i.e., Diff-Quik).

In the cat, mild anemias that are regenerative may have minimal or no polychromasia. The lack of obvious regeneration (reticulocytosis) does not rule out either hemorrhage or hemolysis. Potential causes include early hemorrhage or hemolysis, immune-mediated disease directed at RBC precursors, and recent transfusion, as well as anemia caused by multifactorial causes. If polychromasia is not evident in a feline blood smear, a reticulocyte count is recommended, which is a more accurate way to determine regeneration in cats.

NEXT STEPS: Significant polychromasia may be used to call an anemia regenerative, but the absence of polychromasia should be interpreted cautiously. The anemia may appear nonregenerative in early acute hemorrhagic or hemolytic anemias, and polychromasia may be difficult to recognize with some stains. Thus, if the onset of anemia is unknown, serial complete blood count (CBC) examinations may be needed to evaluate for regeneration. Reticulocyte counts should also be performed in cases where regeneration is questioned.

Plate 2-6   Polychromasia

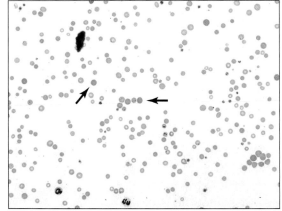 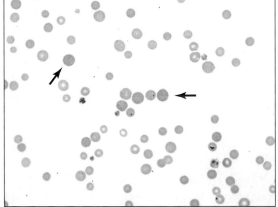

Plate 2-6   Polychromasia *(con't)*

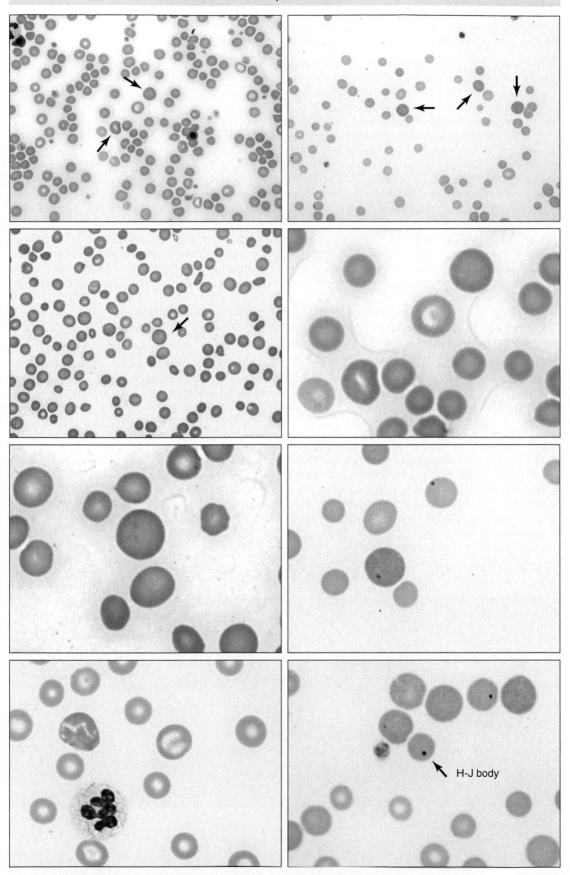

H-J body

Reticulocytes

DISTINCTIVE FEATURES: When immature, anucleate erythrocytes are stained with a supravital stain such as new methylene blue (NMB), the stain penetrates the RBC membrane and binds to the ribosomes, staining them dark blue and causing them to clump, which identifies these cells as reticulocytes.

The dog has only one identifiable form of reticulocytes in peripheral blood, called aggregate *reticulocytes*. Cats, in contrast, have two: (1) punctate reticulocytes and (2) aggregate reticulocytes. Punctate reticulocytes contain few, small, dotlike (punctate), blue-black structures (small polyribosome aggregates) but no large aggregates of ribosomes. Aggregate reticulocytes contain one or more medium to large, blue-black structures that may appear as a cluster or network of aggregated structures.

The clinical usefulness of punctate reticulocyte counts in cats remains unclear. Many laboratories and all hematology instruments that report reticulocyte counts in cats, count and report only aggregate reticulocytes. Manual reticulocyte counts are done by counting the number of reticulocytes present in 1000 RBCs. The percentage is determined by dividing the number of reticulocytes counted by 10. The absolute reticulocyte count is determined by multiplying the reticulocyte % by the RBC count. The degree of reticulocytosis is best indicated by the absolute aggregate reticulocyte count (see the Appendix for more information).

Canine reticulocytes released from the bone marrow mature rapidly from aggregate reticulocytes to mature erythrocytes in approximately 24 hours. Punctate reticulocytes are present in low numbers in dogs. Feline aggregate reticulocytes released from bone marrow mature within 12 to 24 hours to the punctate reticulocyte stage. Feline punctate reticulocytes may take up to 2 weeks to develop into mature erythrocytes.

Usually, good correlation exists between the degree of polychromasia observed on a blood film and the aggregate reticulocyte numbers (with the exception of cats, see above). Punctate reticulocytes appear the same as mature erythrocytes on a Wright-stained blood film.

DIAGNOSTIC SIGNIFICANCE: The effectiveness of bone marrow response to anemia is determined by the number of aggregate reticulocytes in dogs and cats. Regenerative anemias occur secondary to blood loss and IMHA if the bone marrow is healthy. Some heavy metal toxicities, in particular, lead poisoning, result in excessive numbers (relative to the degree of anemia) of reticulocytes and nucleated RBCs (nRBCs). A mild to moderate anemia may be seen typically only in chronic lead poisoning. Also, with lead poisoning, basophilic stippling is noted within mature RBCs stained with Wright stain.

> **NEXT STEPS:** If the anemia is regenerative (above reference interval), top considerations include blood loss (internal or external hemorrhage) or hemolysis. Note that chronic blood loss anemia may be nonregenerative because of iron deficiency. If the anemia is not adequately regenerative, it should be investigated if adequate time has elapsed for a regenerative response to have occurred. If deemed truly nonregenerative, further testing such as biochemical profile, urinalysis, and bone marrow cytology are indicated.

Plate 2-7 Reticulocytes A, Canine B, Feline

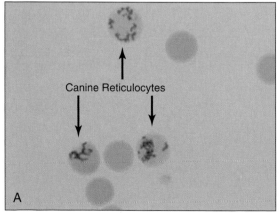

Canine Reticulocytes

A

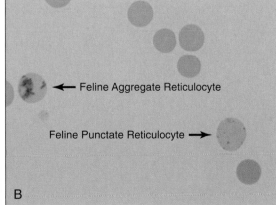

◄— Feline Aggregate Reticulocyte

Feline Punctate Reticulocyte —►

B

Plate 2-7 Reticulocytes *(con't)*

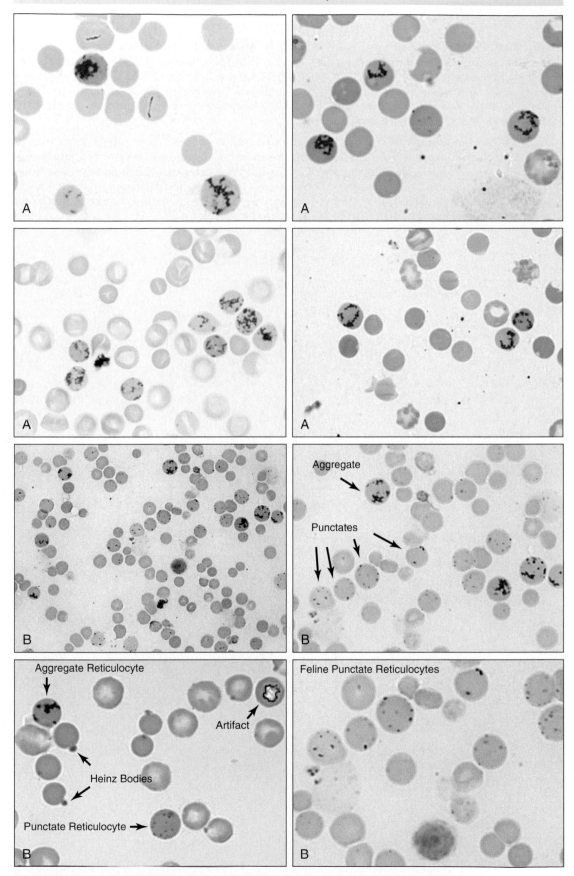

Aggregate

Punctates

Aggregate Reticulocyte

Artifact

Heinz Bodies

Punctate Reticulocyte

Feline Punctate Reticulocytes

Hypochromia

DISTINCTIVE FEATURES: Hypochromic RBCs are excessively pale mature erythrocytes with increased central pallor, showing a gradual change from a pale central area to a light red periphery.

DIAGNOSTIC SIGNIFICANCE: Hypochromic RBCs are hemoglobin deficient mature erythrocytes. Increased hypochromia indicates iron deficiency anemia, which occurs secondary to low-grade, chronic blood loss. Iron deficiency anemia may be secondary to blood loss from the gastrointestinal tract (ulcers, neoplasia, parasites); blood loss in urine (urinary tract infection, calculi, or neoplasia); or external blood loss from blood sucking ectoparasites (fleas, ticks). Milk is low in iron; therefore, young, nursing animals are very susceptible to developing iron deficiency.

NEXT STEPS: Hypochromic RBCs must be differentiated from artifacts. Hypochromic RBCs show a gradual change from red to pale. Artifacts appearing as punched-out centers with a sharp demarcation from dark (red) to light (clear area) are called *torocytes*. Torocytes are artifacts and do not indicate iron deficiency anemia. Dogs often develop hypochromic RBCs with iron deficiency anemia but feline erythrocytes are less likely to become hypochromic. Significant hypochromia warrants ruling out sources of chronic blood loss. An iron profile may also be considered.

Plate 2-8   Hypochromic Red Blood cell

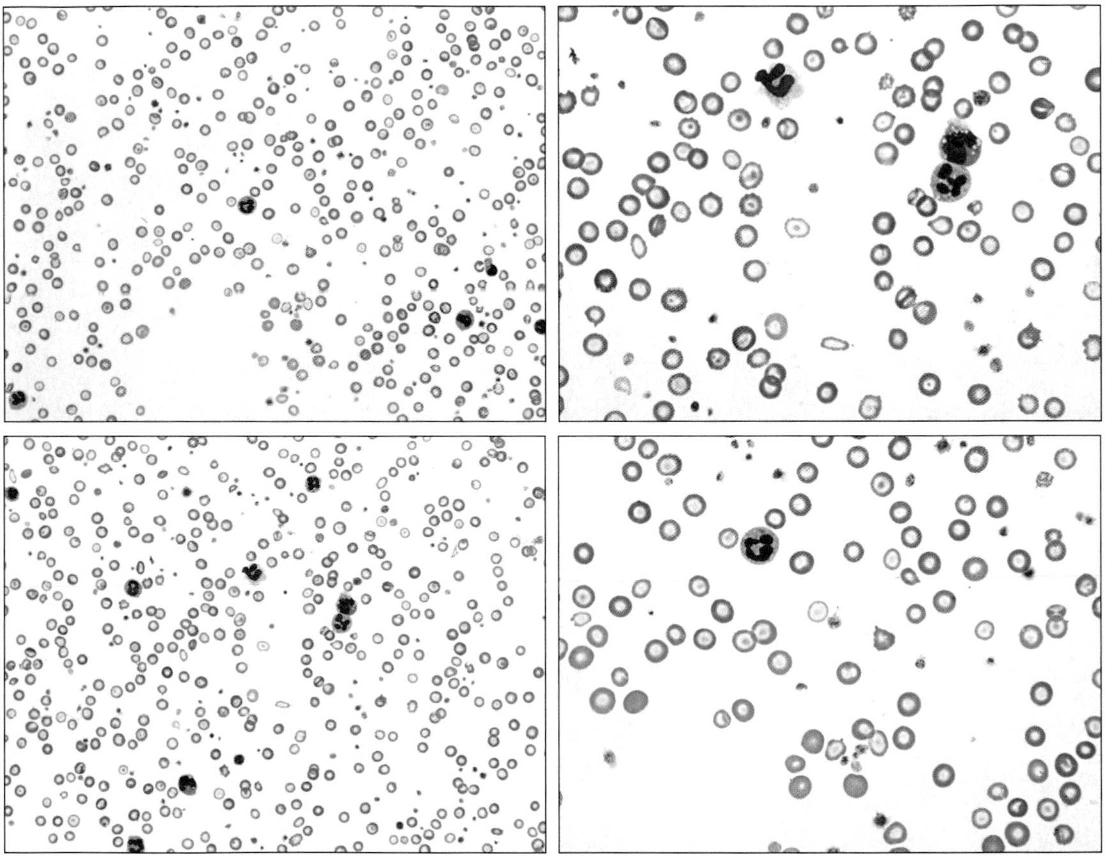

Plate 2-8 Hypochromic Red Blood cell *(con't)*

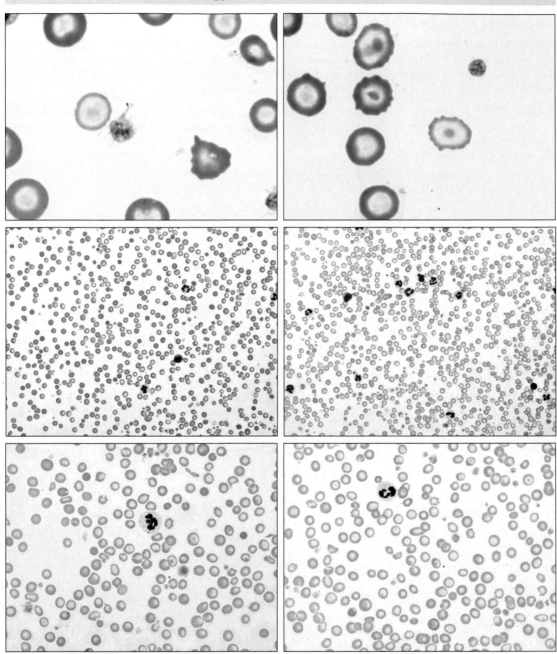

Anisocytosis

DISTINCTIVE FEATURES: Variation in cell size is called anisocytosis. Normal erythrocytes may vary (larger or smaller) up to one third of their size in normal animals.

DIAGNOSTIC SIGNIFICANCE: Increased anisocytosis occurs when significant numbers of small-diameter RBCs, large-diameter RBCs, or a combination of both are present together with normal-diameter RBCs. Anisocytosis is most often recognized with significant numbers of spherocytes in IMHA and large numbers of macrocytic polychromatophils in regenerative anemias.

NEXT STEPS: The significance of anisocytosis is dependent on the numbers of variably sized RBCs and the specific morphology of the RBCs constituting the anisocytosis (i.e., spherocytes, polychromatophils, etc.).

Plate 2-9   Anisocytosis

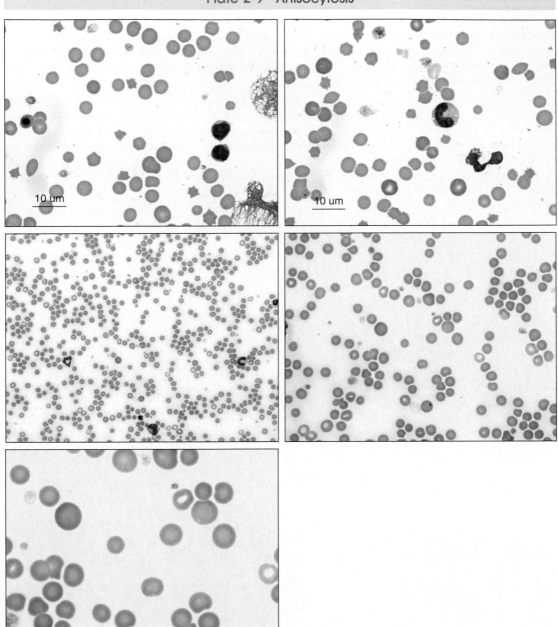

10 um

10 um

Macrocytosis

DISTINCTIVE FEATURES: Macrocytosis is defined as larger than normal RBCs.

DIAGNOSTIC SIGNIFICANCE: Macrocytosis secondary to reticulocytosis is expected in regenerative anemias. Macrocytosis is abnormal when secondary to feline leukemia virus (FeLV) infection in cats (myelodysplastic syndrome, erythroleukemia) or inherited disorders such as macrocytosis of poodles (poodle marrow dyscrasia).

> **NEXT STEPS:** When significant numbers of macrocytic RBCs are evident, investigate for a regenerative anemia (expect concurrent polychromasia). In anemic cats with asynchronous regeneration (i.e., large number of nRBCs and absent or minimal polychromasia or reticulocytosis), consider FeLV testing to aid in identification FeLV associated myelodysplastic syndrome. Check for breed-associated disorders as well. Note that agglutination may cause a falsely increased mean corpuscular volume (MCV), suggesting macrocytosis; as aggregated RBCs are sometimes measured as a single RBC, careful examination of the blood film is important.

Plate 2-10   Macrocytes

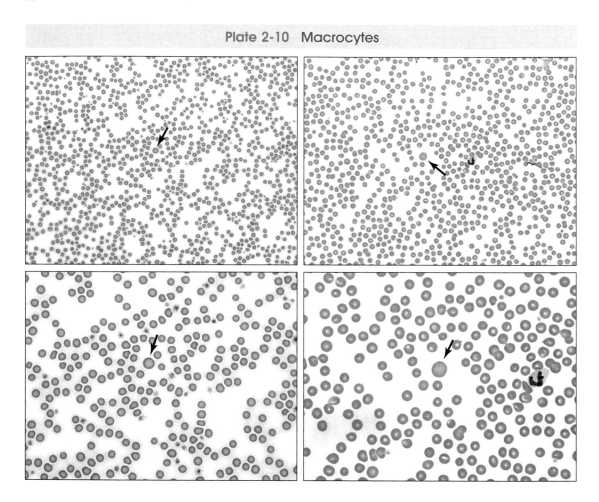

Plate 2-10 Macrocytes *(con't)*

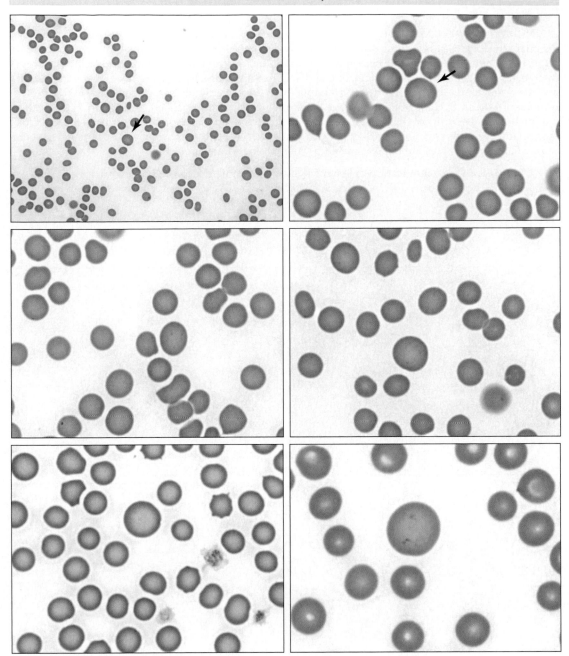

Microcytosis

DISTINCTIVE FEATURES: Microcytes are RBCs with reduced cell volume compared with normal RBCs.

DIAGNOSTIC SIGNIFICANCE: Small RBCs may occur with acquired disorders (i.e., iron deficiency anemia, schistocytosis, bone marrow disorders); congenital disorders (i.e., familial dyserythropoiesis of English Springer Spaniels), and hereditary disorders (i.e., microcytosis of Akita and Shiba Inu dogs). Microcytes may be seen in both congenital and acquired liver disease, in particular liver shunts. MCV may be artifactually low if a short blood sample in an ethylenediaminetetraacetic acid (EDTA) tube is evaluated (excess EDTA). Spherocytes are small-diameter cells, which are included in this section, although these cells are not truly microcytic. Spherocytes may appear as small-diameter cells on a blood smear; however, this is caused by their spheric shape, which conserves volume after removal of membrane. Thus, spherocytes are not considered by many to be true microcytes.

NEXT STEPS: When significant numbers of microcytes are evident on blood smear review, rule out iron deficiency anemia, IMHA, microangiopathy, liver disease, and check for breed-associated disorders.

Plate 2-11   Microcytes

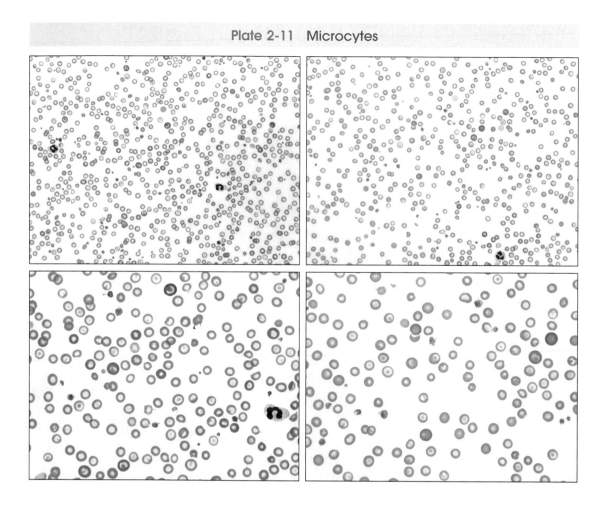

Plate 2-11   Microcytes *(con't)*

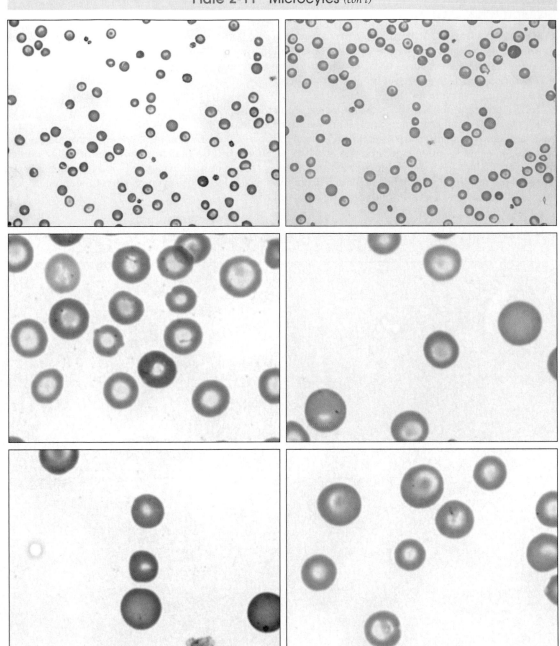

Poikilocytes

DISTINCTIVE FEATURES: Abnormally shaped RBCs are generically termed *poikilocytes*.

DIAGNOSTIC SIGNIFICANCE: Many different forms of poikilocytes exist, as well as many different causes of poikilocytosis; a few important causes include the following:
- In vitro artifactual changes (echinocytes and some acanthocytes)
- RBC fragmentation (schistocytes and keratocytes)
- Membrane loss (spherocytes)
- RBC membrane abnormalities (acanthocytes and stomatocytes)
- Excess RBC membrane compared with cytoplasm (target cells)

The diagnostic significance of poikilocytes depends on which of the many different types are present and, in some cases, is dependent on the numbers of affected RBCs (i.e., low numbers of Heinz bodies may be normally seen in feline blood, but Heinz bodies are not normal in canine blood). Anemia is often associated with poikilocytes and may range from mild to moderate or severe. Some of the more important poikilocytes are discussed individually below.

Plate 2-12   Poikilocytosis

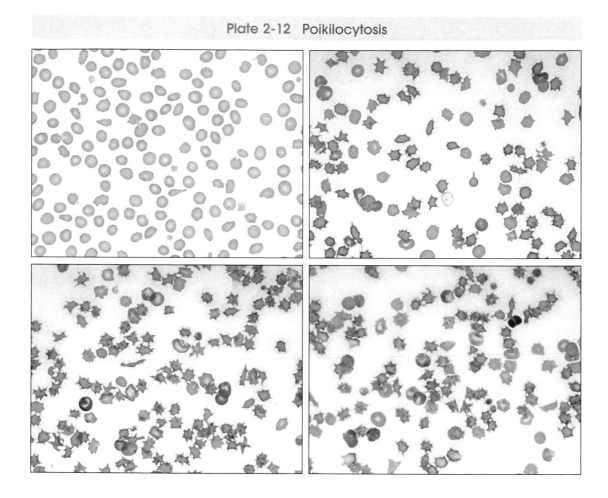

Plate 2-12   Poikilocytosis *(con't)*

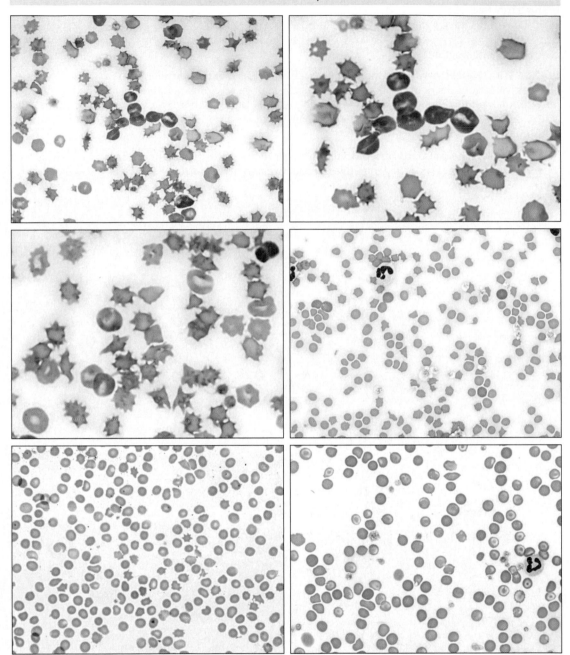

Leptocytes: Target Cells (Codocytes) and Folded Red Blood Cells

DISTINCTIVE FEATURES: Leptocytes are thin erythrocytes and may appear as either target cells or folded cells. Target cells have a dark central area surrounded by a clear area, which is then encircled by a dark peripheral region giving the appearance of a target. Folded cells have a fold in the membrane or have a central bar of hemoglobin.

DIAGNOSTIC SIGNIFICANCE: Occasional target cells are normal in the peripheral blood of dogs. Increased numbers of target cells may be observed in blood from dogs with regenerative anemia, and sometimes, polychromatophilic cells appear as target cells, folded cells, or both. Leptocytes may be seen in pathologic states such as iron deficiency anemia, congenital dyserythropoiesis, liver disease, or nephrotic syndrome.

> **NEXT STEPS:** The presence of leptocytes should prompt investigation into disorders such as iron deficiency anemia, IMHA, regenerative anemia, liver disease, and renal disease.

Plate 2-13   Leptocytes

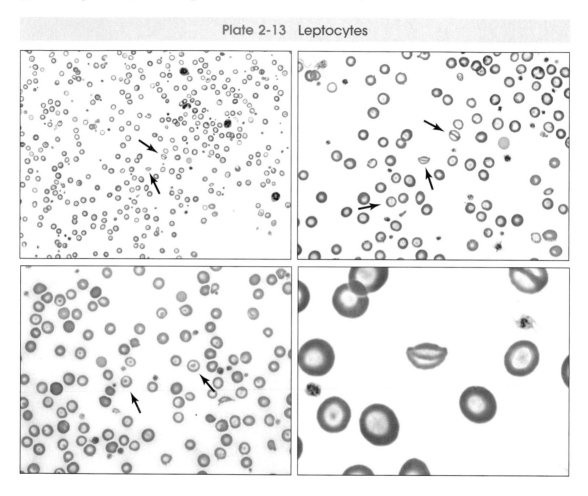

Plate 2-13   Leptocytes *(con't)*

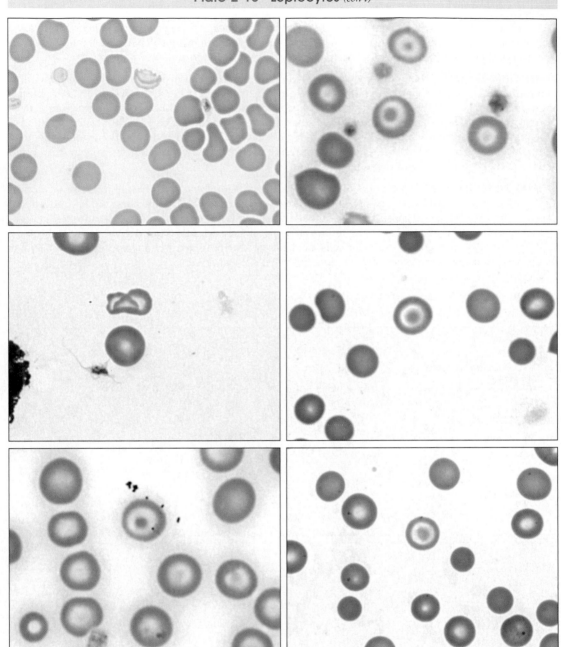

Spherocytes

DISTINCTIVE FEATURES: Spherocytes are small RBCs that are less than two thirds the diameter of normal erythrocytes. As they are spherical and not disc shaped, they lack central pallor and appear dense, often darker (more red in color) than discocytes. Only spherocytes in the monolayer region should be identified, as in other areas of the smear artifactual spherocytes may be present.

DIAGNOSTIC SIGNIFICANCE: Spherocytes are fairly easy to recognize in dogs but are often impossible to recognize in cats, as normal feline RBCs lack central pallor. When spherocytes are observed in moderate to high numbers, IMHA is the most likely cause. IMHA may be a primary (autoimmune mediated) disease or a secondary disease (initiated by primary infectious, inflammatory or neoplastic conditions). Low numbers of spherocytes may be seen in many disorders, including Heinz body hemolytic anemia, hemoparasitism, envenomation (i.e., snake bites and bee stings), zinc toxicity, microangiopathy and neoplasia (i.e., lymphoma and hemangiosarcoma).

NEXT STEPS: If significant numbers of spherocytes are present, look for RBC agglutination to support the diagnosis of IMHA; if agglutination is not evident, consider Coombs test to lend additional support to the IMHA diagnosis. Even if autoagglutination is not evident and the Coombs test is negative, significant numbers of spherocytes are still most likely secondary to IMHA. Carefully check for hemoparasites, circulating neoplastic cells, evidence of neutrophil toxic changes, and other RBC morphologic abnormalities, especially if secondary IMHA is suspected.

Plate 2-14 Spherocytes

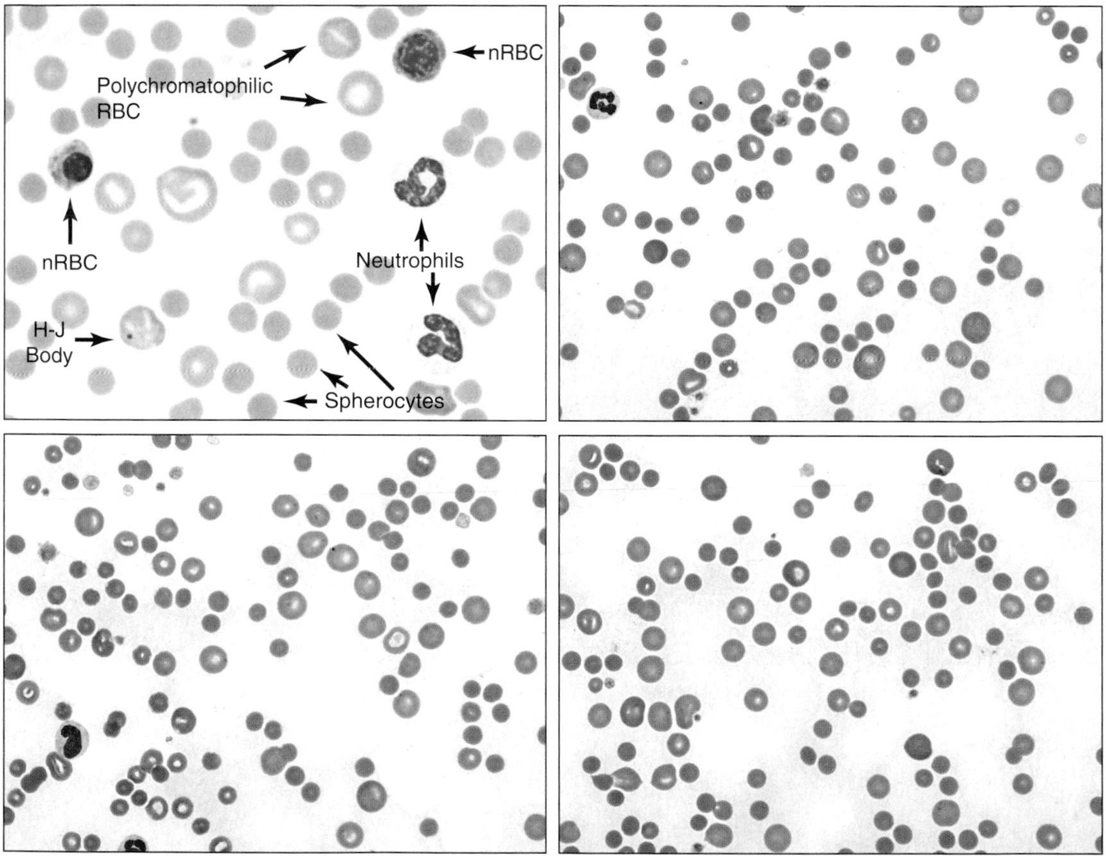

Plate 2-14 Spherocytes *(con't)*

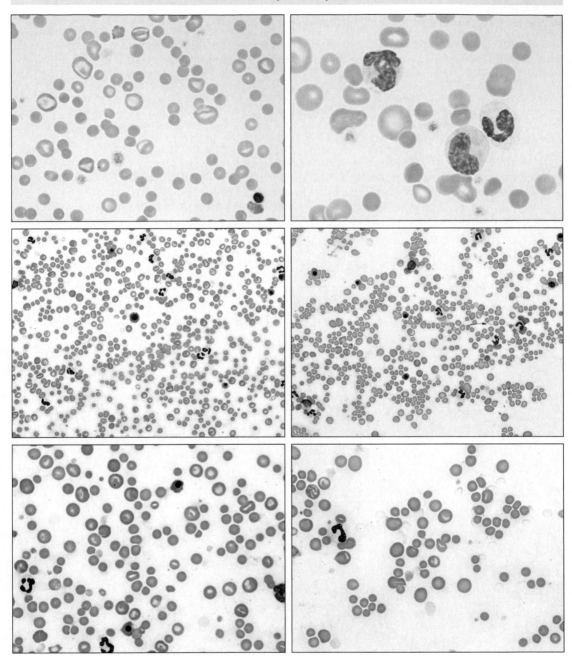

Schistocytes (Fragmented Erythrocytes)

DISTINCTIVE FEATURES: Schistocytes are RBC fragments; they are smaller than normal RBCs, often irregular and sometimes triangular in shape with pointed extremities.

DIAGNOSTIC SIGNIFICANCE: Schistocytes are commonly seen with microangiopathic hemolytic disease, where erythrocytes hit fibrin strands, are cut, and their phospholipid membranes, upon touching, reseal, resulting in circulating erythrocyte fragments.

Schistocytes occur with many disorders such as disseminated intravascular coagulation (DIC), myelofibrosis, vasculitis, glomerulonephritis, hemangiosarcoma, cardiac disease, and iron deficiency anemia. Some of the RBC fragments will round up and become spherocytes; therefore, some spherocytes may be seen along with schistocytes.

NEXT STEPS: Investigate for microangiopathic disease—especially vascular neoplasms of the liver and spleen (hemangiosarcoma). Rule out DIC by evaluating a coagulation profile. To investigate iron deficiency anemia, look for microcytic, hypochromic RBCs and investigate for a source of blood loss (endoparasites, ectoparasites, hematuria, gastrointestinal blood loss). Cardiac auscultation, electrocardiography, heartworm testing, and echocardiography may be considered to assess for cardiac disease.

Plate 2-15   Schistocytes

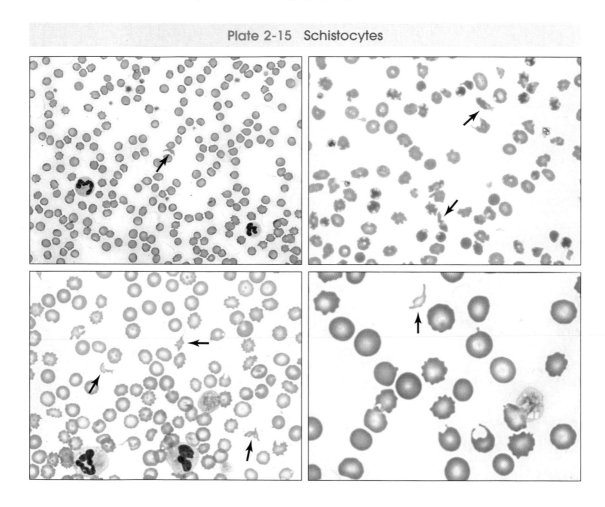

Plate 2-15   Schistocytes *(con't)*

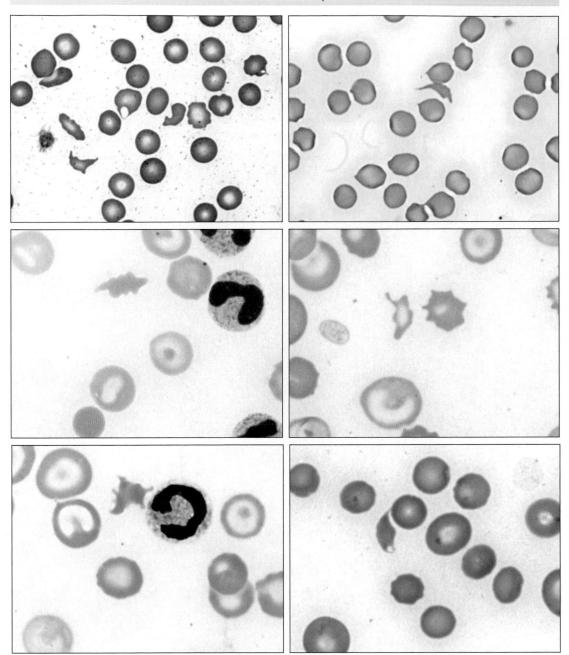

Keratocytes (Blister Cells and Helmet Cells)

DISTINCTIVE FEATURES: Keratocytes are mature erythrocytes that contain single or multiple, intact or ruptured, clear, peripheral circular areas. RBCs containing intact clear circular areas are sometimes called *blister cells*, whereas RBC containing clear circular areas that have ruptured resulting in one or two projections from the RBCs are sometimes called *helmet cells*.

DIAGNOSTIC SIGNIFICANCE: Keratocytes are formed by RBC trauma, very similar to schistocytes. Keratocyte formation is potentiated in feline blood stored in EDTA anticoagulant. Keratocytes are seen in various disorders associated with other RBC abnormalities (i.e., acanthocytosis, echinocytosis) in dogs. Keratocytes may be seen with various other disorders such as DIC, liver disease, vascular neoplasia (i.e., hemangiosarcoma), iron deficiency anemia, and myelodysplastic syndrome.

NEXT STEPS: Many of the same diseases resulting in RBC trauma that form schistocytes also cause keratocyte formation (refer to above section on schistocytes).

Plate 2-16   Keratocytes

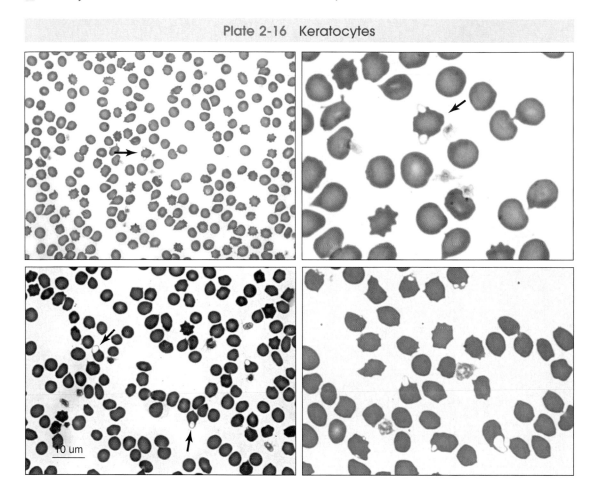

Plate 2-16 Keratocytes *(con't)*

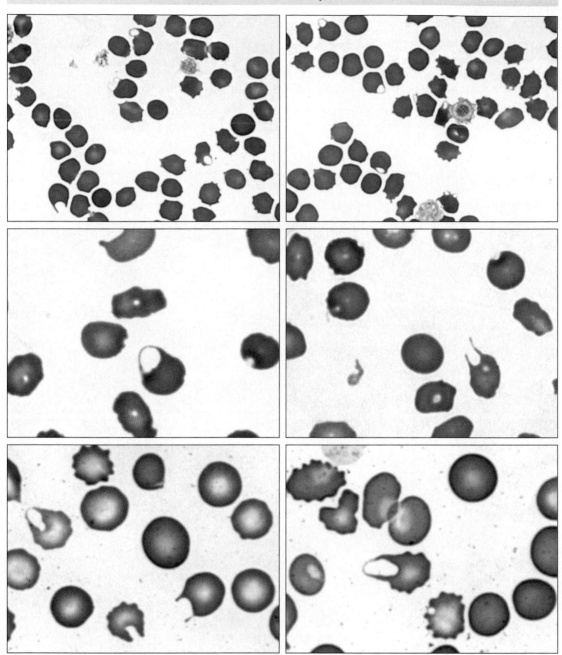

Eccentrocytes (Hemighosts)

DISTINCTIVE FEATURES: Eccentrocytes are mature erythrocytes in which the hemoglobin is pushed to one side of the cell leaving an opposing pale staining region.

DIAGNOSTIC SIGNIFICANCE: Eccentrocytes result from oxidative damage to the erythrocytes from ingestion of exogenous oxidants such as onions, garlic, acetaminophen, propylene glycol (some foods and antifreeze solutions), zinc, and vitamin K antagonist intoxication. They may also be formed from elaboration of endogenous oxidants in some very ill patients with diseases such as diabetes mellitus.

NEXT STEPS: Check for other evidence of oxidative injury to RBCs such as the presence of Heinz bodies. Finding eccentrocytes warrants investigation for oxidant ingestion and for underlying disease.

Plate 2-17   Eccentrocytes

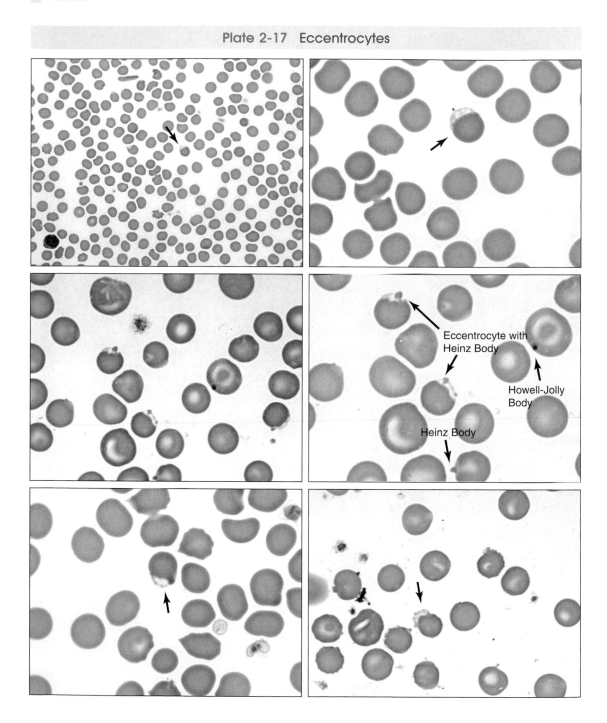

Plate 2-17   Eccentrocytes *(con't)*

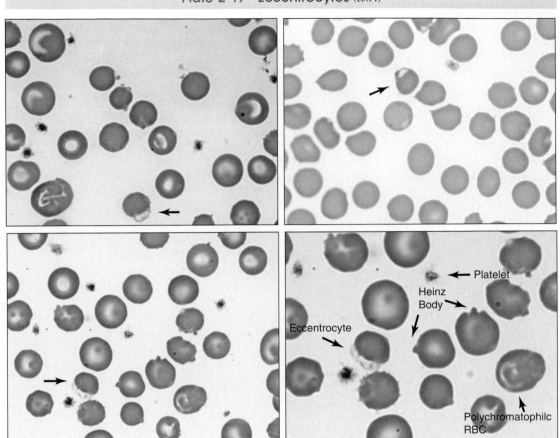

Pyknocytes

DISTINCTIVE FEATURES: Dense, irregularly contracted RBCs are formed by oxidative damage. Pyknocytes look a lot like spherocytes and are often differentiated by the company they keep (i.e., pyknocytes occur with eccentrocytes and may even form from eccentrocytes). Some pyknocytes will have a membranous tag unlike spherocytes, which are smooth and perfectly round. Pyknocytes stain more intensely with NMB stain compared with spherocytes.

DIAGNOSTIC SIGNIFICANCE: Pyknocytes indicate oxidative injury and generally occur with eccentrocytes.

> **NEXT STEPS:** On the basis of history, clinical findings, and laboratory findings, investigate for causes of oxidative insult.

Plate 2-18 Pyknocytes

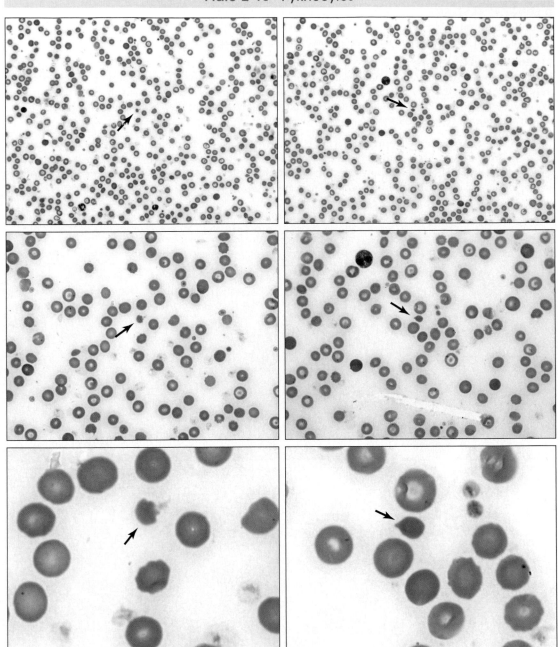

Echinocytes (Crenated Erythrocytes, Burr Cells, Berry Cells)

DISTINCTIVE FEATURES: Echinocytes are spiculated erythrocytes with equally spaced projections over their entire surface. Morphology may vary from irregularly spiculated (type I), to equally spaced blunt projections (type II), to equally spaced pointed projections (type III).

DIAGNOSTIC SIGNIFICANCE: Echinocytes may be an artifact caused by slow drying, excess EDTA, improper smear preparation, or old blood (prolonged storage before smear preparation). However, they may occur secondary to hyponatremic dehydration, renal disease, doxorubicin (a chemotherapeutic) toxicity, certain drugs, and snake bite (rattlesnake and coral snake) and bee sting envenomization, in which the unique type III echinocytes predominate.

> **NEXT STEPS:** When significant numbers of echinocytes are seen, rule out the possibility of an artifact. Make sure these cells are differentiated from acanthocytes (see below). If an artifact is excluded, investigate for patient dehydration and renal disease, review medications, and, if type III echinocytes are evident, rule out snake bite and bee sting envenomation.

Plate 2-19   Echinocytes

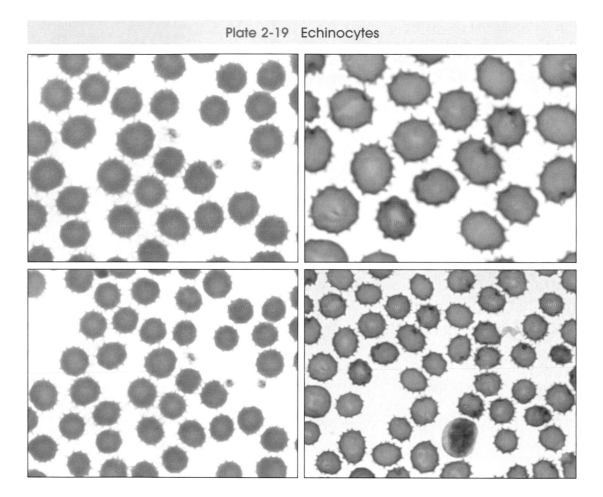

Plate 2-19   Echinocytes *(con't)*

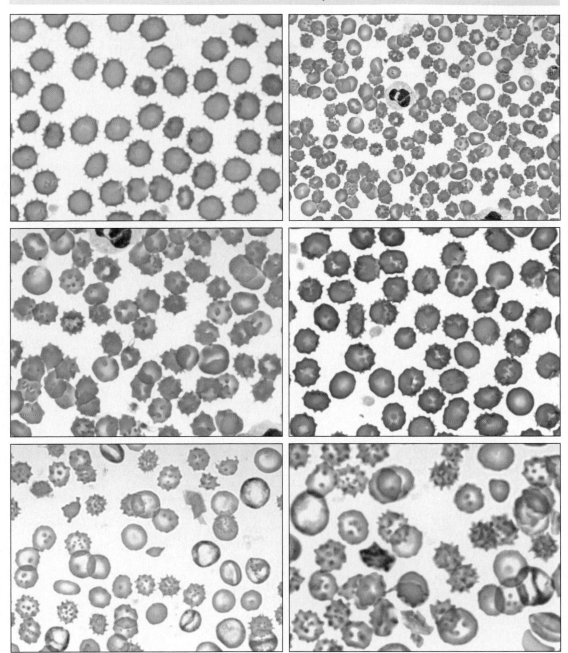

Acanthocytes (Spur Cells)

DISTINCTIVE FEATURES: Acanthocytes are RBCs with multiple, irregular projections that are randomly spaced. Acanthocytes contrast to echinocytes in that acanthocyte projections are randomly spaced, and echinocyte projections are regularly spaced.

DIAGNOSTIC SIGNIFICANCE: Acanthocytes may occur in dogs and cats with liver, splenic, or renal disorders. Acanthocytes are important, as they are often seen in the peripheral blood of patients with vascular neoplasms, in particular hemangiomas and hemangiosarcomas. Acanthocytes may also be seen with DIC and lymphoma.

NEXT STEPS: Make sure to differentiate acanthocytes from echinocytes. If true acanthocytes are present, top considerations include an underlying vascular neoplasm, particularly involving the liver and spleen.

Plate 2-20 Acanthocytes

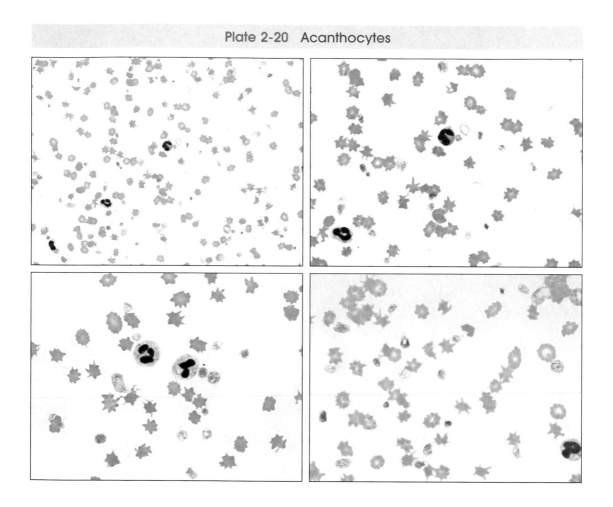

Plate 2-20   Acanthocytes *(con't)*

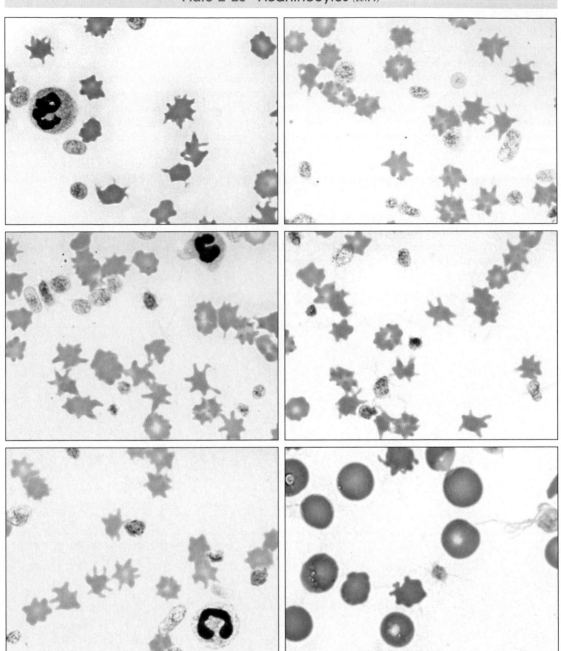

Stomatocytes

DISTINCTIVE FEATURES: Stomatocytes are mature erythrocytes of normal size and color but with an oval or stoma (mouth)–shaped area of central pallor.

DIAGNOSTIC SIGNIFICANCE: Stomatocytes most commonly occur as artifacts, especially in the thick areas of the smear. Stomatocytes occur in high numbers in the peripheral blood of Alaskan Malamutes with hereditary stomatocytosis. This condition is characterized by short-limb dwarfism, chondrodysplasia, and anemia. The erythrocytes have a shortened life span, and a regenerative response is usually evident. Hereditary stomatocytosis has also been reported in Miniature and Standard Schnauzers without clinical signs of disease. Familial stomatocytosis–hypertrophic gastritis is a multiorgan disease affecting Drentse Partirjshond dogs (Dutch Partridge dogs). In Abyssinian and Somali cats, a hereditary RBC defect, characterized by increased osmotic fragility, macrocytosis, and some stomatocytosis, is the suspected cause of recurrent Coombs-negative hemolytic anemia. Small-diameter stomatocytes (termed *imperfect spherocytes* and *stomatospherocytes*) may be seen with some forms of IMHA, particularly those that are poorly regenerative.

NEXT STEPS: When stomatocytes are evident in significant numbers, first investigate for breed-associated disorders. If imperfect spherocytes or stomatospherocytes are evident, assess for other evidence to support the diagnosis of IMHA (i.e., RBC agglutination, ghost RBC, positive Coombs test, RBC regeneration).

Plate 2-21 Stomatocytes

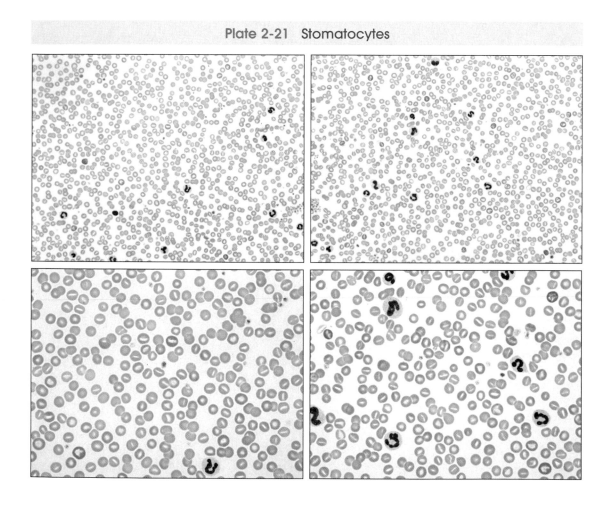

Plate 2-21   Stomatocytes *(con't)*

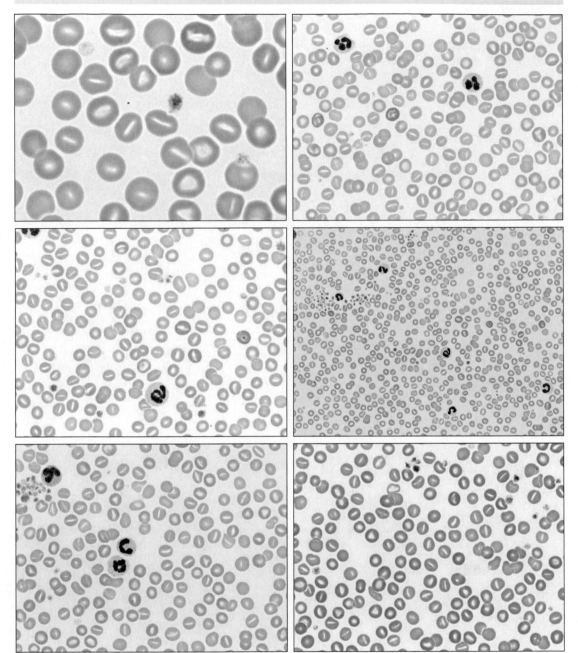

Crystallized Hemoglobin

DISTINCTIVE FEATURES: Large, diamond, rhomboid, rectangular, or square-shaped, intensely staining hemoglobin crystals are observed within RBCs.

DIAGNOSTIC SIGNIFICANCE: Hemoglobin crystals are seen most commonly in cats and rarely in dogs. No recognized significance has been reported.

Plate 2-22   Crystallized Hemoglobin

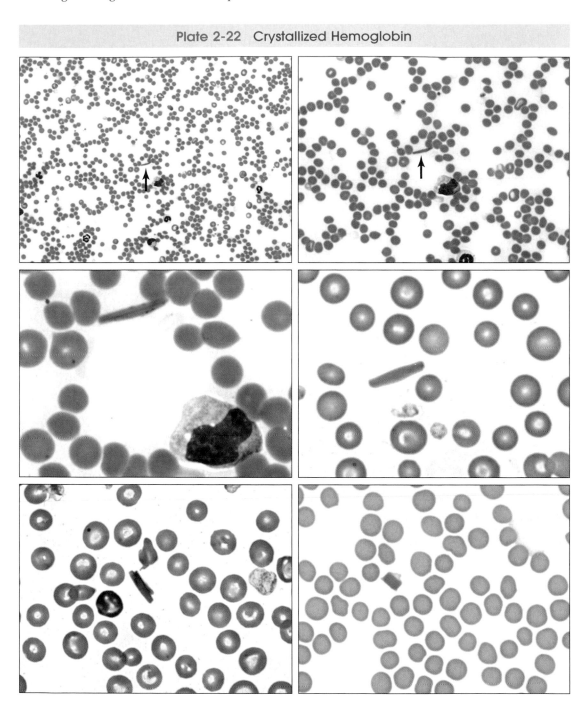

Plate 2-22 Crystallized Hemoglobin *(con't)*

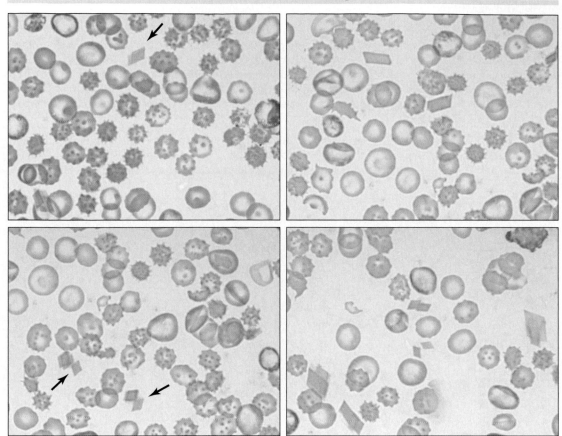

Erythrocytic Ghosts (Lysed Red Blood Cells, Fading Erythrocytes)

DISTINCTIVE FEATURES: Erythrocytic ghosts are pale RBC membranes with no or minimal hemoglobin.

DIAGNOSTIC SIGNIFICANCE: With intravascular hemolysis, the hemoglobin is dispersed, and the erythrocyte membrane is rapidly cleared. Therefore, the presence of erythrocytic ghosts on peripheral blood smears suggests either very recent intravascular hemolysis or in vitro hemolysis. RBC lysis that occurs during smear preparation usually appears as RBC smudges. With lipemia, erythrocytes have increased membrane permeability and fragility, resulting in occasional smudged erythrocytes and erythrocytic ghosts, especially when smears are not made immediately. Smudged erythrocytes are characterized by fuzzy, ill-defined cell borders.

NEXT STEPS: When ghost RBCs are present, evaluate the smear for concurrent RBC agglutination and spherocytosis to lend support to the diagnosis of intravascular hemolysis. Check the specimen for lipemia, and rule out in vitro hemolysis by reviewing blood collection and handling techniques.

Plate 2-23   Erythrocytic Ghosts

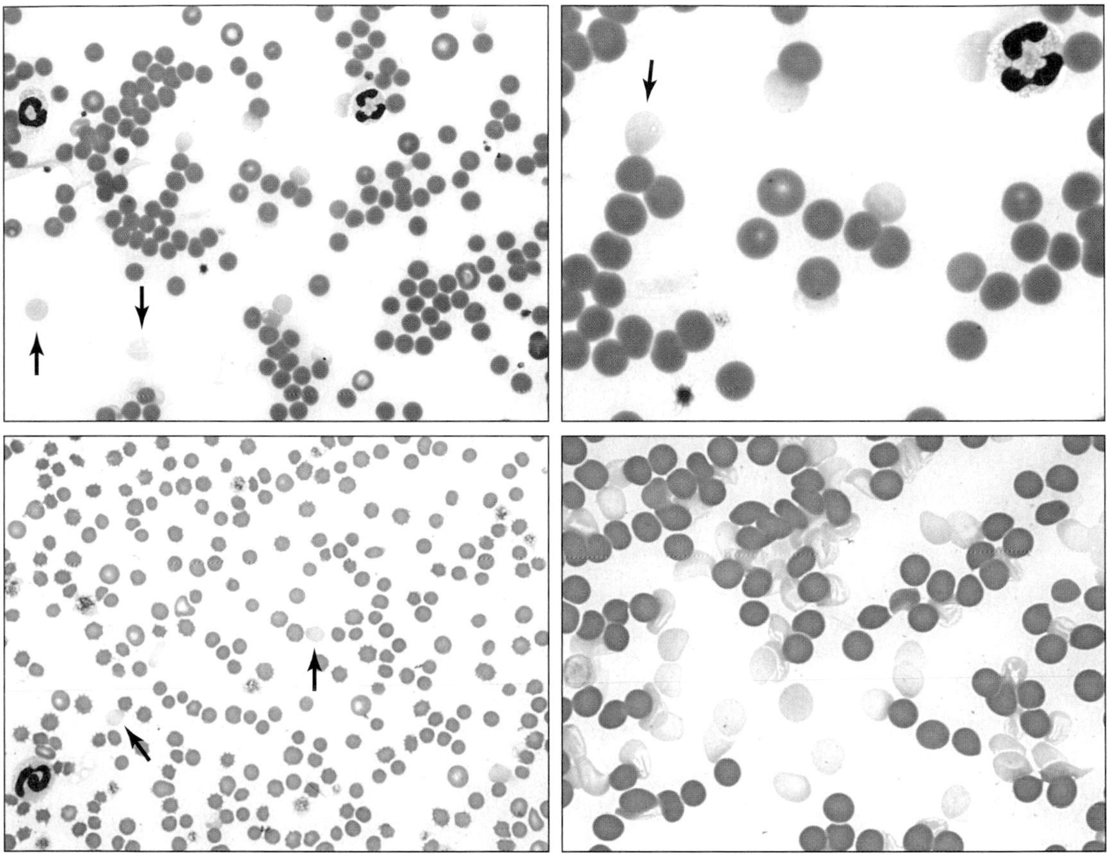

Plate 2-23 Erythrocytic Ghosts *(con't)*

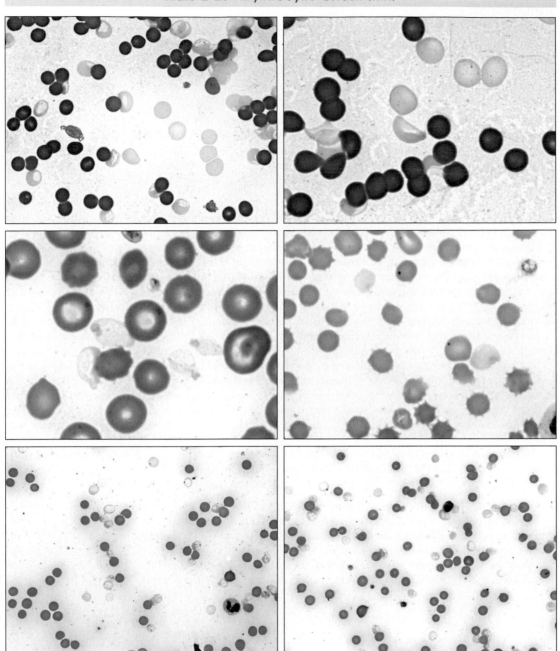

Nucleated Red Blood Cells (Metarubricytes and Rubricytes)

DISTINCTIVE FEATURES: Metarubricytes and rubricytes are nRBCs that are most commonly seen in peripheral blood smears. These cells have small, round, central nuclei with coarse chromatin (rubricyte) or smooth pyknotic chromatin (metarubricyte), and either polychromatophilic (blue-gray) or orthochromic (orange-red) cytoplasm, which help in differentiating them from small lymphocytes. Additionally, nuclei in nRBCs are central in location, and a rim of cytoplasm may be traced around the entire nucleus. In contrast, it is difficult to trace a complete rim of cytoplasm around the nucleus of mature lymphocytes because of the eccentric placement of the nucleus.

DIAGNOSTIC SIGNIFICANCE: Nucleated RBCs (usually of the metarubricyte or rubricyte stages) are occasionally found in small numbers in peripheral blood smears from normal dogs and cats (<2 nRBCs/100 WBCs). Nucleated RBCs are quantitated during the WBC differential count, and reported as the number of nRBCs per 100 WBCs. Increased numbers of nRBCs may occur with both regenerative (expected) and nonregenerative anemias (abnormal, suggesting an asynchronous regenerative response).

The most common cause of increased nRBCs is with regenerative anemia (hemorrhage or hemolysis). It is important to note that the presence of nRBCs alone should not be taken as an indication of bone marrow response to an anemia, as increased nRBCs may be seen in nonregenerative anemias. Evaluation of the regenerative response to an anemia should always be based on the degree of reticulocytosis.

Nucleated erythrocytes may be present in low numbers in peripheral blood smears secondary to conditions such as splenic contraction; splenic disease or dysfunction or splenectomy (decreased nRBC removal from the circulation); trauma (bone fractures resulting in immature cells of the marrow entering the circulation); hyperadrenocorticism (Cushing's disease); steroid administration (increased RBC survival time in the circulation); and cardiovascular disease (secondary to hypoxia). They may be seen in certain canine breeds (miniature Schnauzers and toy and miniature Poodles) and in some inflammatory conditions.

Nucleated erythrocytes may be present in low, moderate, or high numbers with many disease states such as regenerative anemias, lead poisoning, bone marrow diseases, hemangiosarcoma, septicemia, and endotoxic shock. Bone marrow neoplasia (primary leukemia or metastatic neoplasia), inflammatory diseases, lead poisoning, and heat stroke may damage the bone marrow sinusoidal endothelial lining and put pressure on marrow hematopoietic tissue, causing nRBCs to more easily and more rapidly pass into the circulation.

More immature stages of nRBCs (back to the rubriblast stage) may be found with some myeloproliferative diseases such as erythroleukemia and sometimes in markedly regenerative anemias, the latter sometimes observed in cats with *Mycoplasma hemofelis* infection.

NEXT STEPS: The significance of finding nRBCs on blood smear review is based on the numbers of nRBCs, ruling out breed differences, and determining if anemia is present. As the differential WBC count is performed, nRBCs are recorded as "nRBCs/100 WBC." If greater than 5 nRBCs/100 WBC are present, most laboratories correct the WBC count for the presence of nRBCs. Some laboratories report the total nucleated cell count, which includes leukocytes and nRBCs. Nucleated RBCs are not included in the differential WBC count, and an absolute number is given.

Plate 2-24   Nucleated Red Blood Cells (nRBCs)

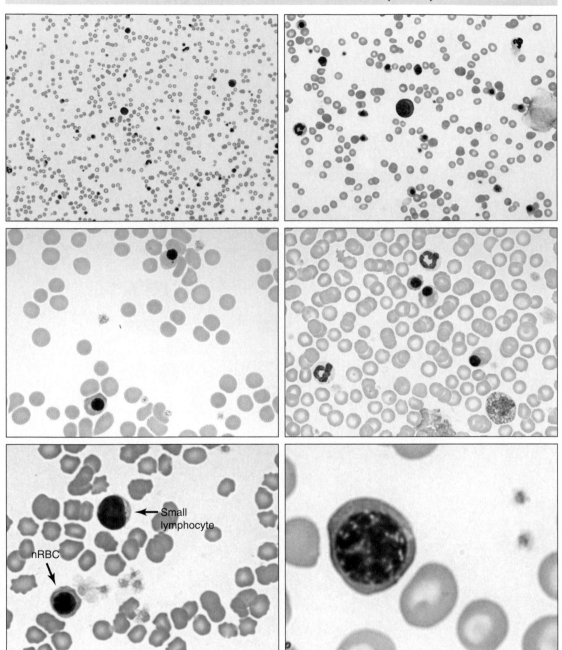

Plate 2-24   Nucleated Red Blood Cells (nRBCs) *(con't)*

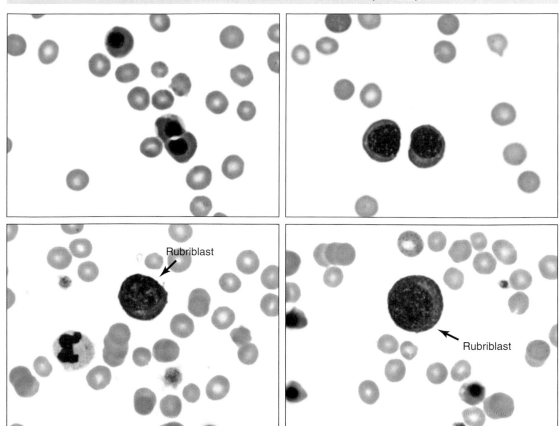

Make sure not to confuse small lymphocytes (**A** and **B**) with nucleated red blood cells (**C** and **D**).

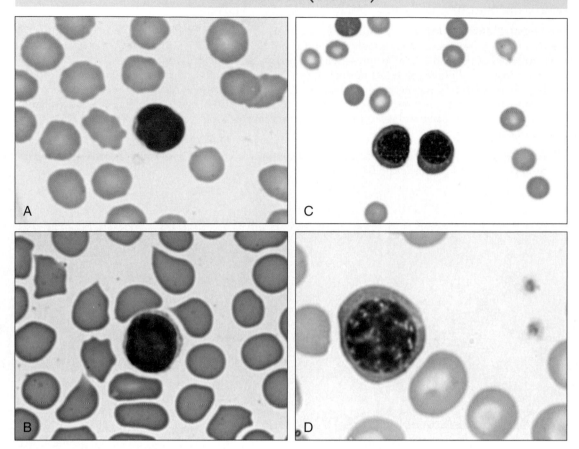

Howell-Jolly Bodies

DISTINCTIVE FEATURES: Howell-Jolly bodies (H-J bodies) are small, homogeneous, dark purple (same color as RBC nuclei), spherical structures within the RBC cytoplasm.

DIAGNOSTIC SIGNIFICANCE: H-J bodies are fragments of RBC nuclei retained after expulsion of the nucleus (nuclear remnants). One should be careful not to confuse H-J bodies with an erythroparasite. Low numbers of H-J bodies may be present in the peripheral blood of normal cats and are infrequently observed in the peripheral blood of normal dogs. The number of erythrocytes containing H-J bodies tends to increase during regenerative anemias (similar to the increase in nRBCs) as well as other conditions (similar disorders and mechanisms seen with increased nRBCs) such as splenic disease, postsplenectomy state, bone marrow disease (myelophthesis), chemotherapy, radiation, erythroid toxins, and glucocorticoid therapy.

NEXT STEPS: The number of H-J bodies and association with anemia or normovolemia determine the significance of H-J bodies found on blood smear review.

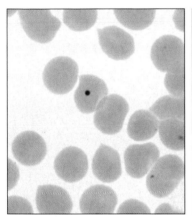 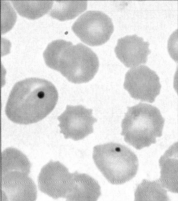 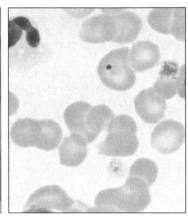

Plate 2-25   Howell-Jolly Bodies

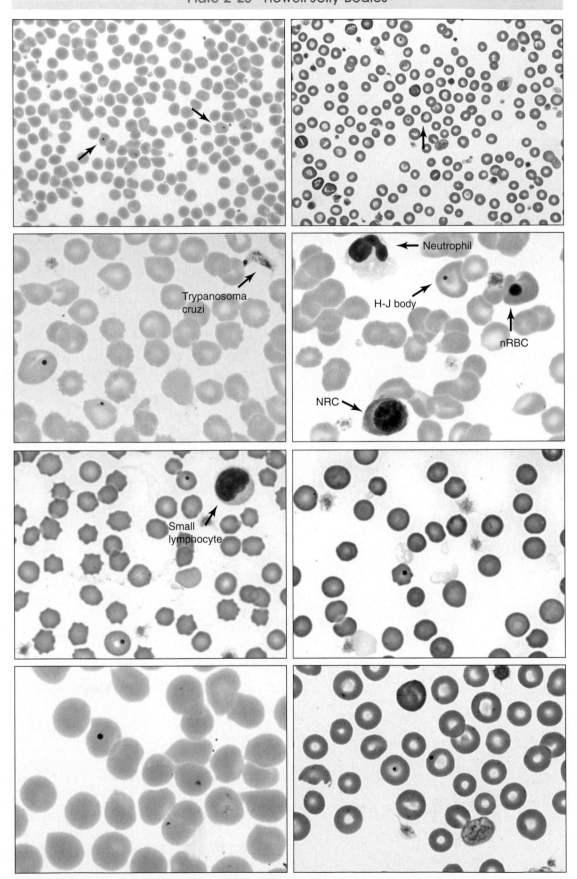

Make sure not to confuse Howell-Jolly bodies with: **A,** *Babesia gibsoni*
B, Canine Distemper Inclusions **C,** Basophilic stippling

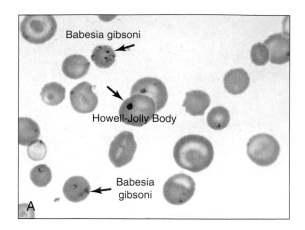

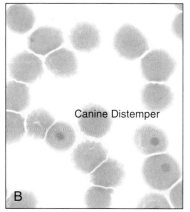

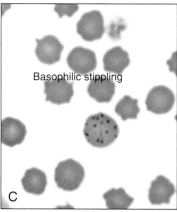

Make sure not to confuse Howell-Jolly bodies with: **D,** Cytauxzoon felis

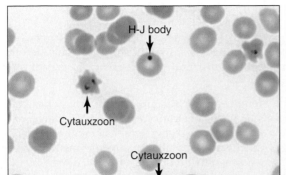

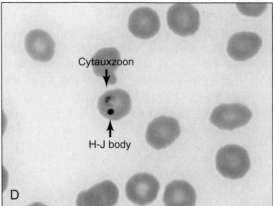

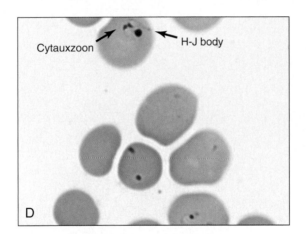

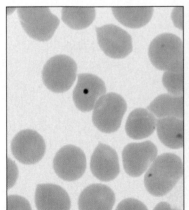

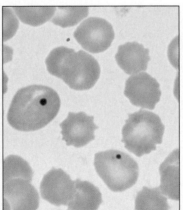

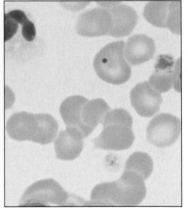

Basophilic Stippling

DISTINCTIVE FEATURES: When ribosomes become unstable, aggregate, and precipitate during drying of the blood film, they stain as faint blue-black dots evenly dispersed within erythrocytes and are recognized as basophilic stippling.

DIAGNOSTIC SIGNIFICANCE: Basophilic stippling may occur with regenerative anemias in both dogs and cats and commonly with lead poisoning. Make sure to distinguish basophilic stippling from siderotic inclusions (see below). Basophilic stippling is usually finely distributed throughout the cytoplasm, whereas siderotic inclusions tend to aggregate loosely.

> **NEXT STEPS:** If basophilic stippling and moderate numbers of nRBCs are present in a nonanemic patient or in one with a mild anemia, blood lead levels should be determined to rule out lead toxicosis. Mild anemia may occur with chronic lead exposure. Assess for neurologic signs, gastrointestinal clinical signs, or both, which occur secondary to lead poisoning. If basophilic stippling (primarily within polychromatophilic RBCs) is evident with a strongly regenerative moderate or marked anemia, the basophilic stippling is likely secondary to erythroid regeneration.

Plate 2-26   Basophilic Stippling

Make sure to distinguish basophilic stippling from Pappenheimer bodies
(see Section II, plate 27, for illustrations of Pappenheimer bodies).

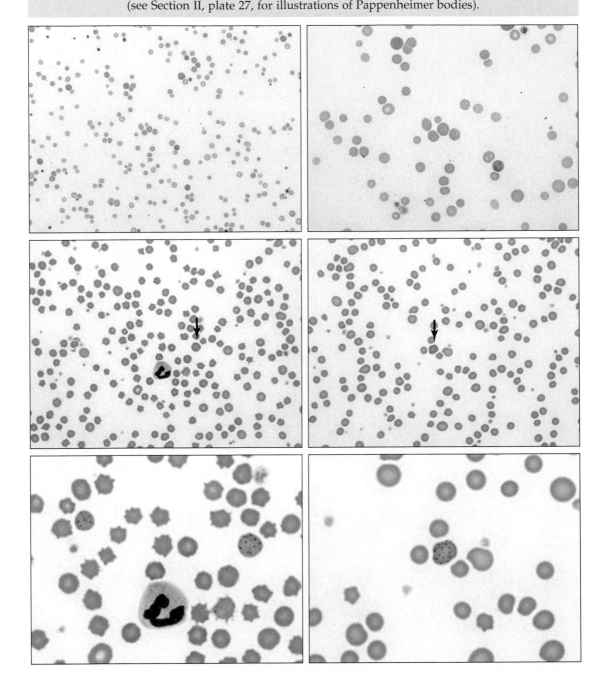

Plate 2-26 Basophilic Stippling *(con't)*

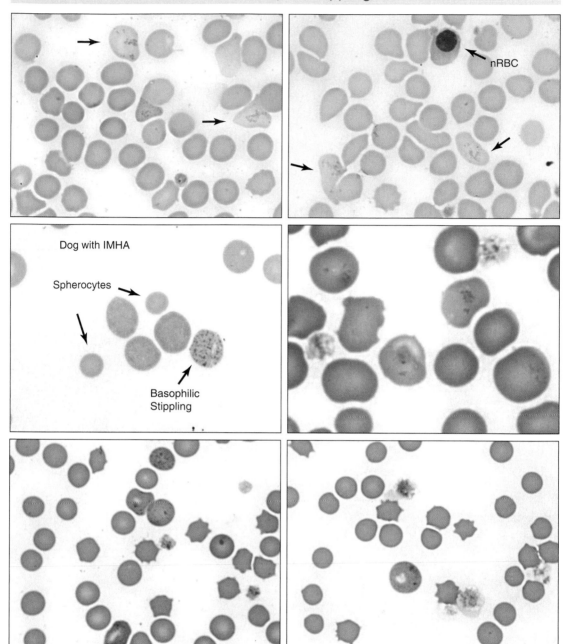

Make sure not to confuse with basophilic stippling. **A,** Canine distemper inclusions **B,** Howell-Jolly bodies **C,** Babesia gibsoni

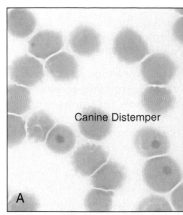

Canine Distemper

A

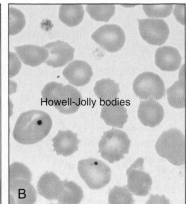

Howell-Jolly bodies

B

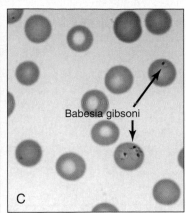

Babesia gibsoni

C

Siderotic Inclusions (Pappenheimer Bodies)

DISTINCTIVE FEATURES: Siderotic inclusions are aggregated basophilic structures generally eccentrically placed on one side near the periphery of the RBC.

DIAGNOSTIC SIGNIFICANCE: These are iron-containing inclusions that are occasionally seen in disorders such as lead poisoning, hemolytic anemia, dyserythropoiesis, and myeloproliferative disorders. Polychromatophilic RBCs and mature RBCs containing these inclusions are called *siderocytes*.

NEXT STEPS: Distinguish siderotic inclusions from basophilic stippling (see section on basophilic stippling). If evidence of lead poisoning is present (mild to no anemia, basophilic stippling, and increased numbers of nRBCs), blood lead levels should be determined. If signs of dyserythropoiesis or myeloproliferative disease are evident on blood film evaluation, examination of a bone marrow sample may be indicated. While seldom done, a Prussian blue stain can be used to confirm the presence of Pappenheimer bodies (siderotic inclusions will stain blue).

Plate 2-27   Siderotic Inclusions

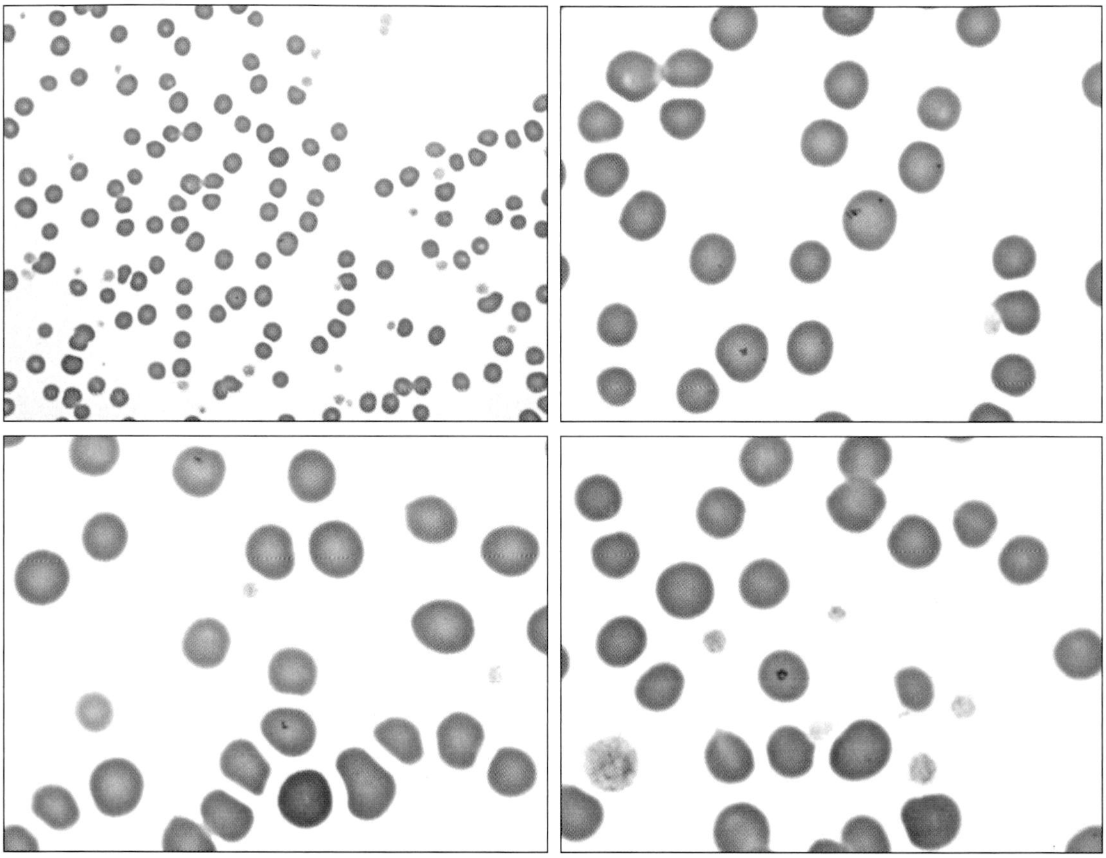

Plate 2-27   Siderotic Inclusions *(con't)*

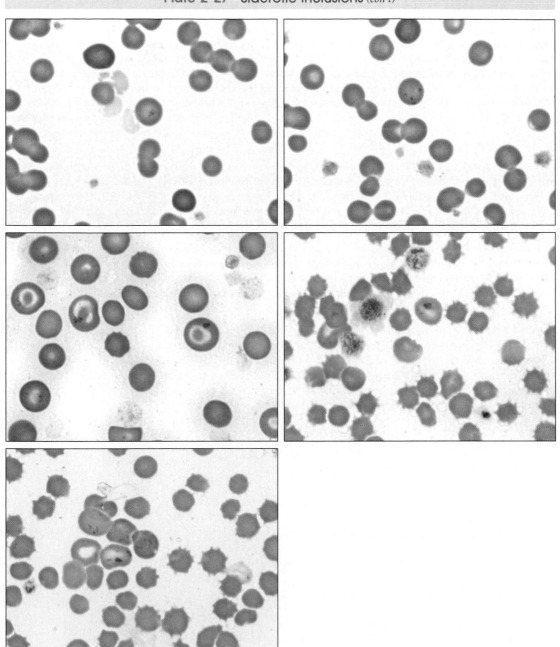

Heinz Bodies

DISTINCTIVE FEATURES: Heinz bodies appear as singular, round projections from the RBC membrane. They may be quite small or very large and prominent. In some cases, a single RBC may have several small Heinz bodies. Heinz bodies stain the same red-pink color of mature RBCs with routine Wright stains, and stain pale basophilic with Diff-Quik stain. With Diff-Quik stain, Heinz bodies may be seen both as round projections from the RBC membrane and as clear round inclusions that have not yet projected out from the RBC membrane. If the presence of Heinz bodies is in question, or to get a more accurate determination of the number of Heinz bodies present, a blood smear may be stained with NMB. With NMB, Heinz bodies stain blue-black, whereas the RBC is pale aqua. In wet mount preparations with NMB, Heinz bodies appear as refractile inclusions when out of focus and are sometimes referred to as *erythrocyte refractile bodies (ER bodies)*.

DIAGNOSTIC SIGNIFICANCE: Heinz bodies occur from oxidative injury resulting in denatured (oxidized), precipitated hemoglobin that tends to adhere to the inner surface of RBC membranes. Heinz bodies are seen most frequently in peripheral blood smears from cats (up to 5% of RBC in normal cats have small Heinz bodies). Feline RBCs are more susceptible to Heinz body formation, and the feline spleen is nonsinusoidal and less efficient at removing Heinz bodies.

Large numbers of Heinz bodies are seen in sick cats, especially those with diabetes mellitus, hyperthyroidism, and lymphoma. Heinz bodies are always abnormal in dogs. Some causes of Heinz body hemolytic anemia secondary to oxidant ingestion include onions, garlic, acetaminophen, methylene blue, methionine, phenazopyridine, zinc (pennies minted after 1982), naphthalene (chemical in mothballs), propylene glycol (in some moist foods), and vitamin K_3 (menadione).

NEXT STEPS: If moderate to high numbers of Heinz bodies are present in feline blood smears or any Heinz bodies are detected in canine blood, first rule out oxidant ingestion. In cats, rule out underlying metabolic disease (diabetes mellitus and hyperthyroidism) and lymphoma. Both enumeration of Heinz bodies and assessment of the size of the Heinz bodies are useful in determining the extent of oxidative injury. Also, carefully check RBC morphology for the presence of eccentrocytes, pyknocytes, and ghost RBCs, which may also be seen with oxidative RBC damage.

Plate 2-28   Heinz Bodies

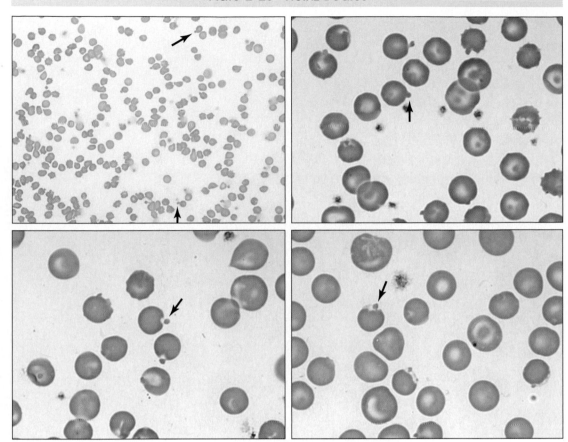

Plate 2-29   Pale Staining Heinz bodies

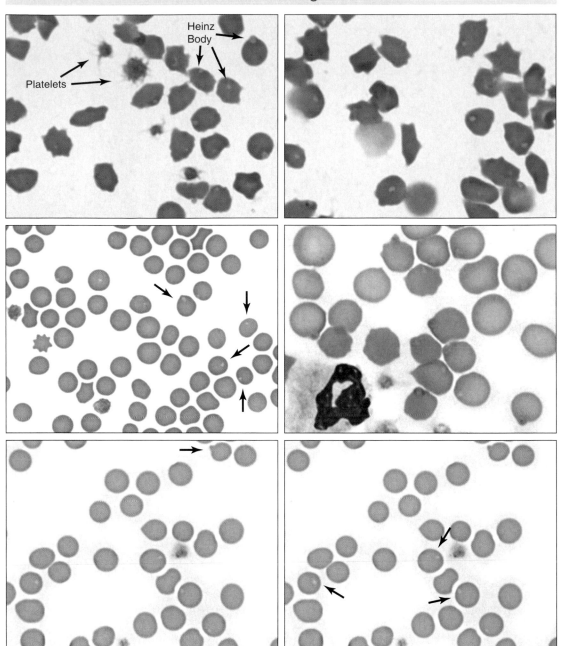

Plate 2-30   Heinz Bodies Stained with New Methylene Blue (NMB)

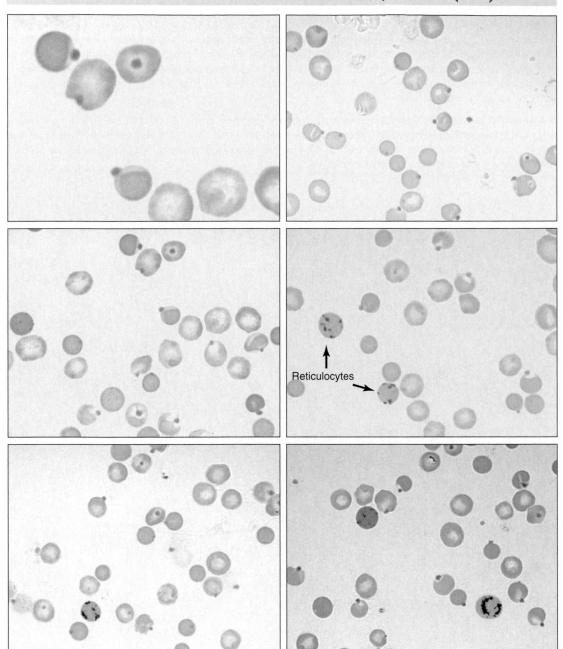

Reticulocytes

Distemper Inclusions

DISTINCTIVE FEATURES: Distemper inclusions are aggregates of viral nucleocapsids that appear microscopically as round to oval to irregular, red to blue inclusions. The inclusions tend to occur in either the monocyte and lymphocyte cell series or the neutrophil and erythrocyte cell series. However, in some cases of distemper, all cell lines may have inclusions. Distemper inclusions are most easily identified on Diff-Quik–stained smears, where the inclusions stain a bright, homogeneous eosinophilic color. Distemper inclusions may be seen on Wright's-stained smears; however, they tend to stain pale blue and are more difficult to identify.

DIAGNOSTIC SIGNIFICANCE: Distemper inclusions are seen only rarely on peripheral blood smears from dogs with distemper infection; however, when present, they are diagnostic for infection. Inclusions are found in a small percentage of dogs during the viremic phase of distemper, which is usually associated with clinical signs of upper respiratory disease.

Plate 2-31   Distemper Inclusions **A.** Diff-Quick–stained **B.** Wright's stained

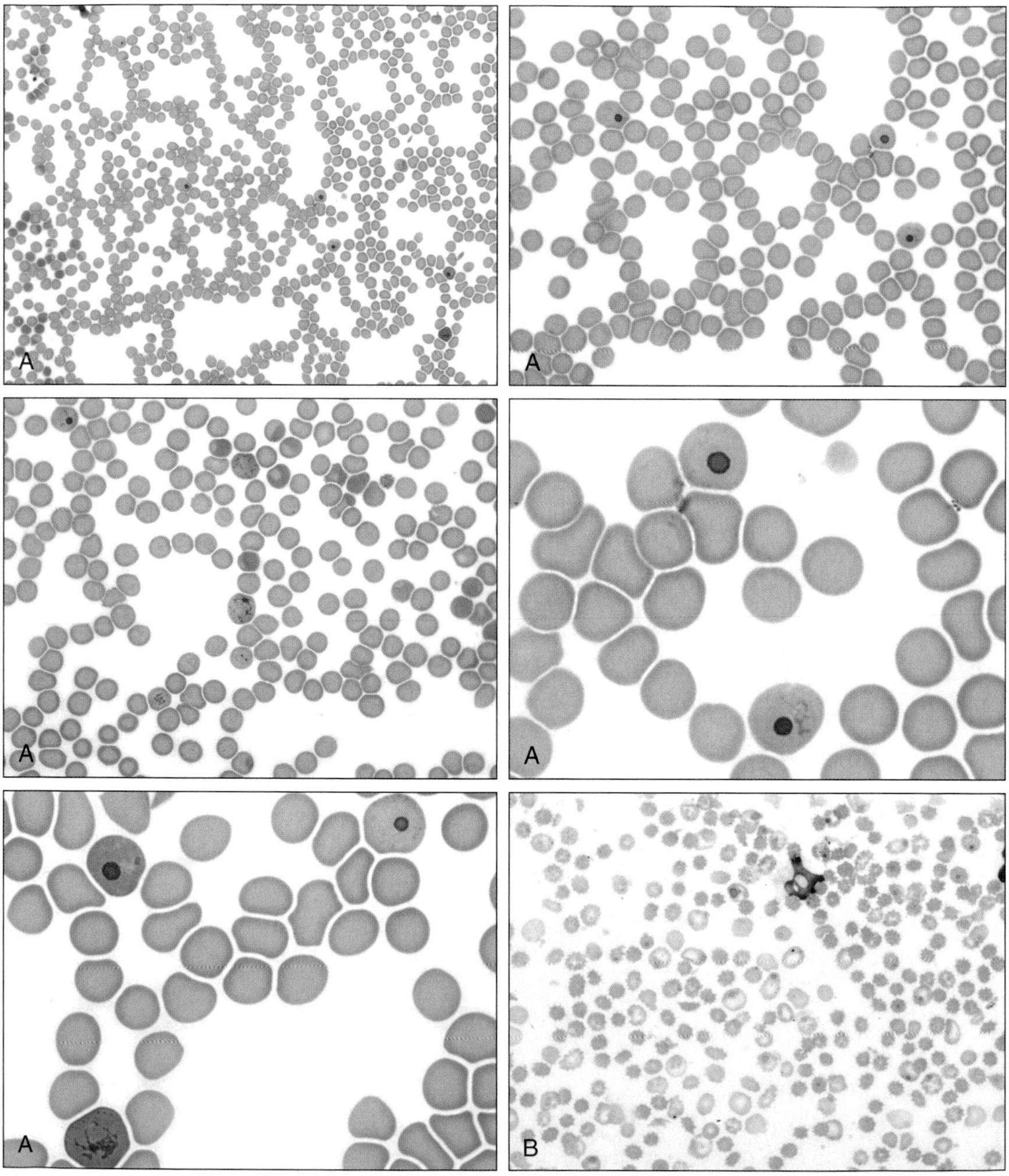

Plate 2-31   Distemper Inclusions *(con't)*

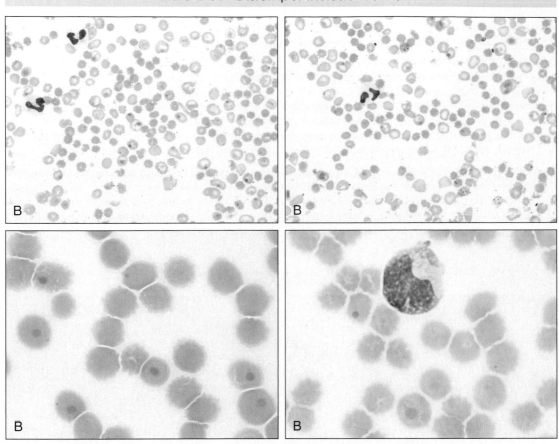

Make sure not to confuse Distemper inclusions with **A,** Basophilic stippling **B,** Howell-Jolly bodies **C,** Babesia gibsoni

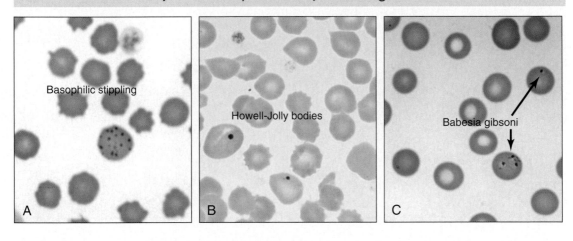

Dysplastic Changes

DISTINCTIVE FEATURES: Dysplastic changes of the erythroid cell line may include large RBCs, maturation asynchrony (fully hemoglobinized RBCs with retained nuclei), binucleate nRBCs, and nRBCs with fragmented nuclei and megaloblasts (extremely large nRBCs).

DIAGNOSTIC SIGNIFICANCE: Very mild erythroid dysplasia may occur in markedly regenerative states and is associated with accelerated hematopoiesis. The most significant dysplastic changes are found with myelodysplastic syndromes (MDSs), notably with FeLV-induced myelodysplasia in cats. Myelodysplastic syndromes are associated with cytopenia(s) and ineffective hematopoiesis with evidence of cellular dysplasia in peripheral blood and bone marrow. Often, an asynchronous regenerative response to the anemia exists, as polychromatophilic RBCs or reticulocytes are infrequent to absent, yet increased nRBCs are present. Some MDSs have evidence of dysplasia in the myeloid and platelet cell lines as well.

NEXT STEPS: When dysplastic nRBCs are found, if the changes are mild and infrequent, and a significant, markedly regenerative anemia exists, then, this is likely secondary to accelerated hematopoiesis. Note that dysplasia may occur secondary to some disease states, toxins, and drugs. If erythropoiesis is ineffective and many significant dysplastic changes have occurred, bone marrow cytology is advised to confirm MDS. In cats, FeLV testing should be performed as well.

Plate 2-32   Dysplastic Changes

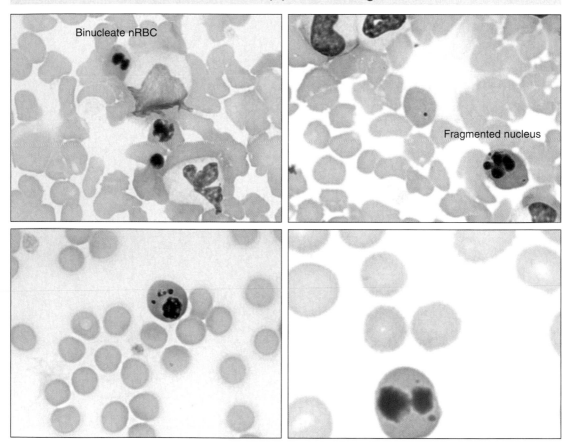

Binucleate nRBC

Fragmented nucleus

Plate 2-32 Dysplastic Changes *(con't)*

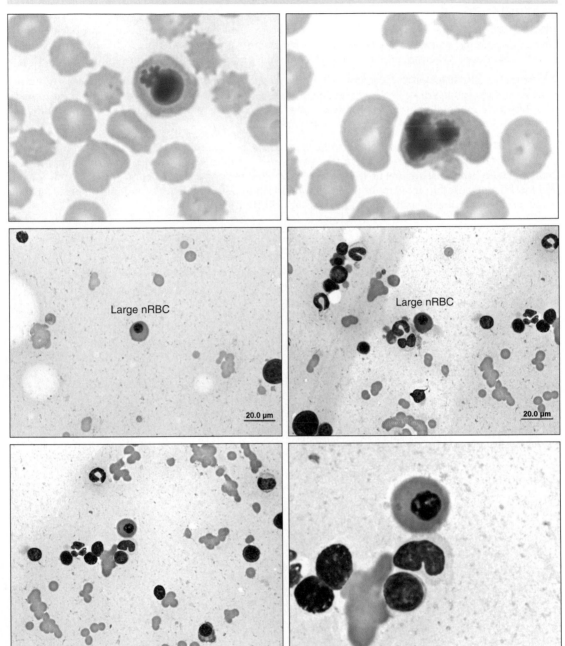

Erythrocytic Parasites

Mycoplasma hemocanis (*previously* Hemobartonella canis)

DISTINCTIVE FEATURES: *Mycoplasma hemocanis (Hemobartonella canis)* organisms are gram-positive parasites of dogs found on the surface of the RBC and generally appear as blue-black, filamentous chains of small rods or dots. When found on the blood smear, the organisms are often present in high numbers.

DIAGNOSTIC SIGNIFICANCE: Infection with *Mycoplasma hemocanis* typically only causes significant disease in dogs that have been splenectomized, have severe splenic disease, or are immunocompromised and thus have moderate to severe hemolytic anemia. Occasional spherocytes and positive Coombs test suggest an immune-mediated component to the anemia.

> **NEXT STEPS:** If the patient is known to be splenectomized, antibiotic treatment is warranted. If the patient is not splenectomized, assessment for disease of the spleen or causes of immunosuppression along with antibiotic treatment is recommended. Polymerase chain reaction (PCR) testing on the blood may be used to confirm infection by identification of the presence of organism-specific nucleic acid (deoxyribonucleic acid [DNA], ribonucleic acid [RNA]).

Plate 2-33 *Mycoplasma hemocanis*

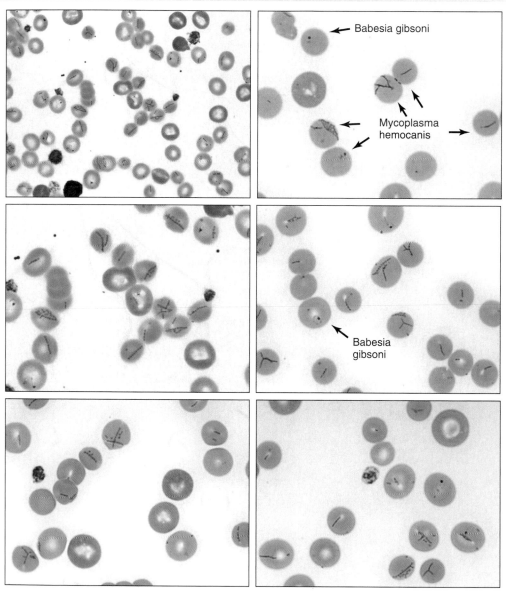

Plate 2-33   *Mycoplasma hemocanis* (con't)

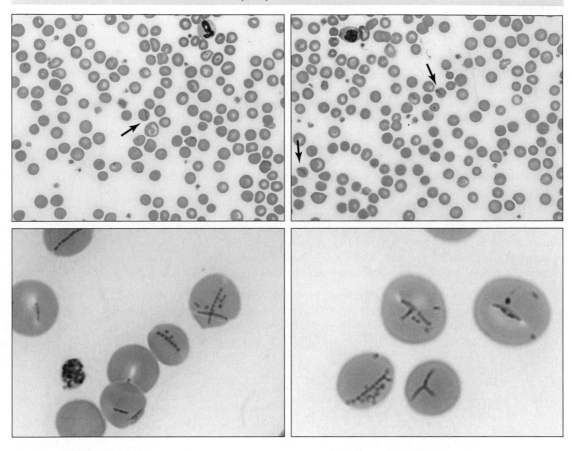

Make sure not to confuse Mycoplasma hemocanis with **A,** Stain precipitate **B,** Extracellular bacteria

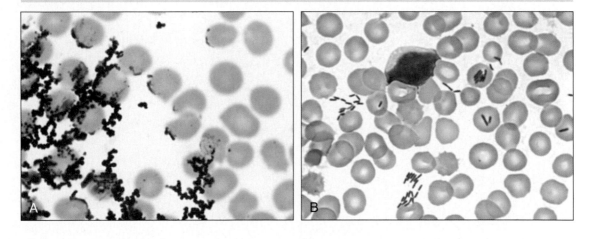

Mycoplasma hemofelis *(previously* Hemobartonella felis*)*

DISTINCTIVE FEATURES: *Mycoplasma hemofelis (Hemobartonella felis)* organisms are gram-positive, epicellular parasites of cats. The organisms form small dots or rods on the surface of the RBC. They stain blue-black and tend to occur on the periphery of erythrocytes. Occasional chains of dots and ring forms may be seen.

DIAGNOSTIC SIGNIFICANCE: Infection with *Mycoplasma hemofelis* may be primary or secondary. Primary disease results in an acute, moderate to severe anemia with a marked regenerative response. As in dogs with *M. hemocanis* infection, an immune-mediated component to the anemia may exist (autoagglutination and positive Coombs test). Many cats are subclinically infected, and the parasitemia is only recognized when the patient becomes immunocompromised by another disease process (i.e., neoplasia, FeLV infection) resulting in secondary disease. In these cases, the anemia is often nonregenerative or poorly regenerative. Some of the most severe anemias occur with concurrent FeLV and *Mycoplasma* infection. Note that not finding *Mycoplasma* organisms during a routine slide evaluation does not rule out the possibility of infection.

Mycoplasma organisms are present on the outside of the erythrocyte; therefore, blood smears should be made soon after blood collection, as the parasites may dislodge from the erythrocyte membrane. In this case, the organisms may be found free in the extracellular space on blood films but are extremely difficult to distinguish from stain precipitate. Thus, if confirmation of the parasite is sought from an outside consultant, premade blood smears should be submitted along with an EDTA tube of whole blood.

NEXT STEPS: If *Mycoplasma* organisms are confirmed on blood smear review, antibiotic treatment is warranted. If suspected, PCR testing for *Mycoplasma* species is recommended. Rule out concurrent disease (i.e., neoplasia, FeLV, and FIV infection) and check the blood film for autoagglutination of RBC to rule out a concurrent immune-mediated component to the anemia.

Plate 2-34 *Mycoplasma hemofelis*

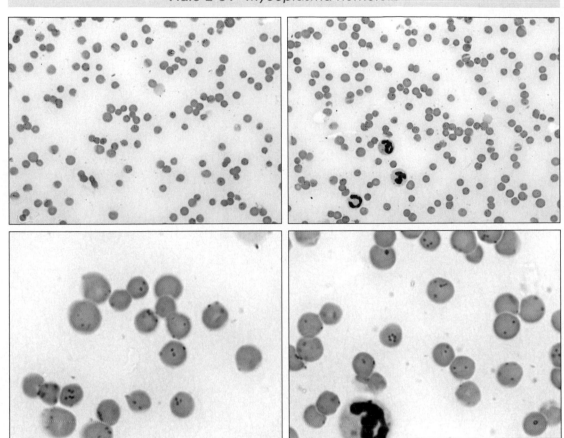

Plate 2-34   *Mycoplasma hemofelis* *(con't)*

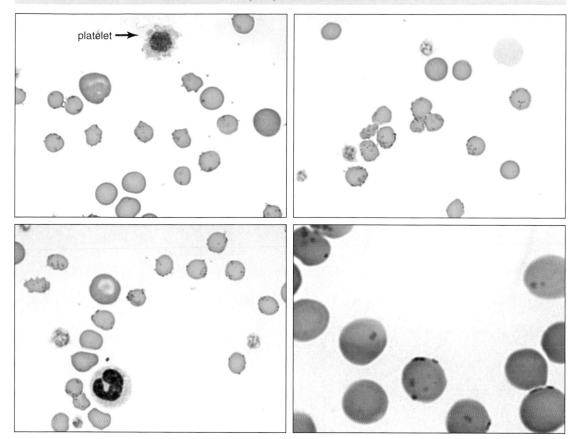
platelet

Plate 2-34 *Mycoplasma hemofelis* *(con't)*

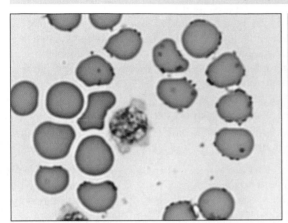

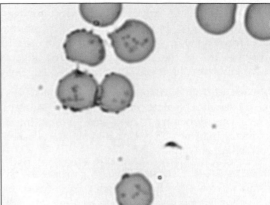

Make sure not to confuse *Mycoplasma hemofelis* with **A,** stain precipitate **B,** extracellular bacteria

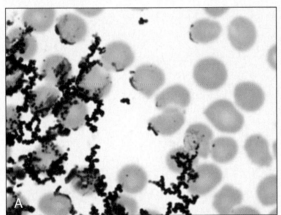

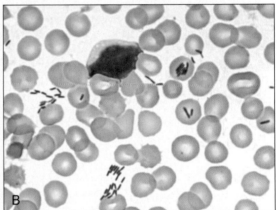

Cytauxzoon felis

DISTINCTIVE FEATURES: *Cytauxzoon felis* is a protozoal hemoparasite of the cat and is readily identified by its "signet ring" appearance. Lower numbers of "safety pin" and "Maltese cross" forms may be observed. *Cytauxzoon felis* is an intraerythrocytic parasite that is generally present in only a small percentage (approximately 1%) of erythrocytes. In the terminal stages of the disease, organisms may be present in up to 25% of the erythrocytes. Rarely, large macrophages containing schizonts full of developing merozoites are observed on the feathered edge of the blood smear.

DIAGNOSTIC SIGNIFICANCE: Cytauxzoonosis is a highly fatal disease of domestic cats. Nonfatal forms have been identified in some parts of the country. The severe clinical signs (depression, fever, anorexia, icterus) are secondary to the tissue phase of infection (infection of the spleen, liver, lung, lymph nodes, and bone marrow). The associated anemia is usually nonregenerative, and concurrent thrombocytopenia and leukopenia may exist.

NEXT STEPS: *Cytauxzoon felis* organisms are differentiated from *Mycoplasma hemofelis* on peripheral blood smears by finding signet ring–shaped organisms with generally a single organism per erythrocyte, as opposed to finding multiple, dot- or rod-shaped organisms on the periphery of the RBC, respectively.

Plate 2-35 *Cytauxzoon felis*

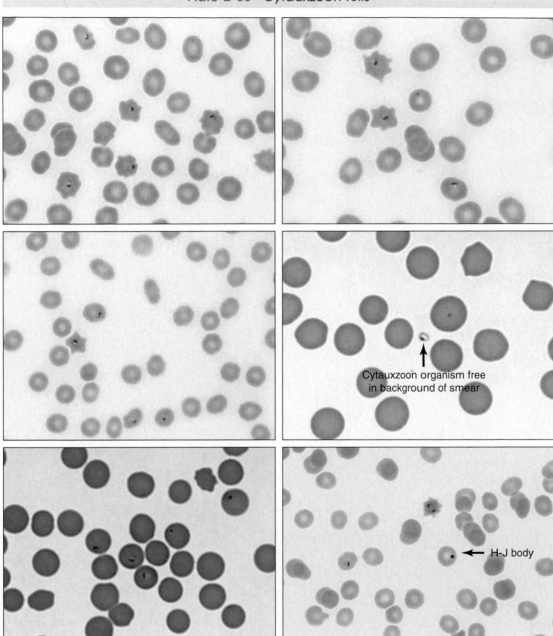

Cytauxzoon organism free
in background of smear

H-J body

Plate 2-35 *Cytauxzoon felis* (con't)

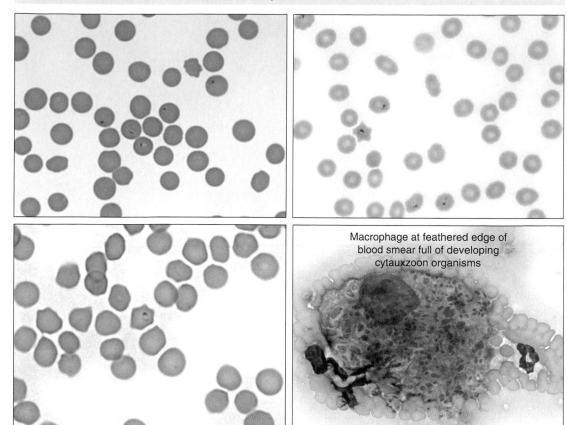

Macrophage at feathered edge of blood smear full of developing cytauxzoon organisms

Make sure not to confuse *Cytauxzoon felis* organisms with Howell-Jolly (H-J) bodies

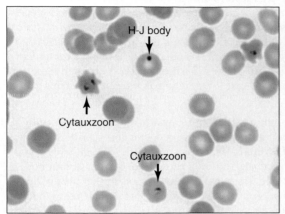

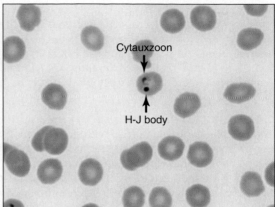

Babesia *spp.*

DISTINCTIVE FEATURES: *Babesia* organisms are intraerythrocytic protozoal parasites. In dogs, two forms are distinguished by size: (1) *Babesia canis* are large organisms that appear as singular or paired piroplasms and may be oval, pear shaped, or ovoid. Currently, three subspecies of *Babesia canis* (subspecies: *canis, vogeli,* and *rossi*) have been identified. The different subspecies have variable virulence, with clinical signs ranging from mild to severe. The second form of *Babesia* organisms are small and form single to multiple signet rings within infected RBCs. To date, three main species of small *Babesia* have been identified: (1) *B. gibsoni,* (2) *B. conradae,* and (3) *B. microti*–like piroplasms (*Theileira annae*). With both large and small *Babesia,* the organism's cytoplasm tends to stain clear to blue, whereas the nucleus stains red to purple.

DIAGNOSTIC SIGNIFICANCE: *Babesia* organisms are intracellular and cause hemolytic anemia with an intravascular component, often with a concurrent thrombocytopenia. Spherocytes and a positive Coombs test may indicate an immune-mediated component. Primary babesiosis generally results in a strongly regenerative anemia. In some animals, the infection is subclinical until the animal becomes immunosuppressed with another disease. In the later circumstance, the anemia may be nonregenerative. Clinical signs of babesiosis range from subclinical to mild to severe. Acute disease is often associated with signs of depression, fever, weakness, lymph node enlargement, splenic enlargement, and anemia.

NEXT STEPS: The presence of intraerythrocytic *Babesia* organisms on blood smear review is diagnostic for canine babesiosis. The absence of organisms does not rule out infection that may be subclinical. The two general categories of *Babesia,* the large and small forms, may be identified microscopically. However, further categorization of species and subspecies may only be performed by using molecular techniques (PCR and DNA sequencing).

When *Babesia* organisms are identified, review the blood film carefully for evidence of concurrent IMHA (RBC agglutination and spherocytes), and assess for thrombocytopenia as well.

Plate 2-36 *Babesia canis*

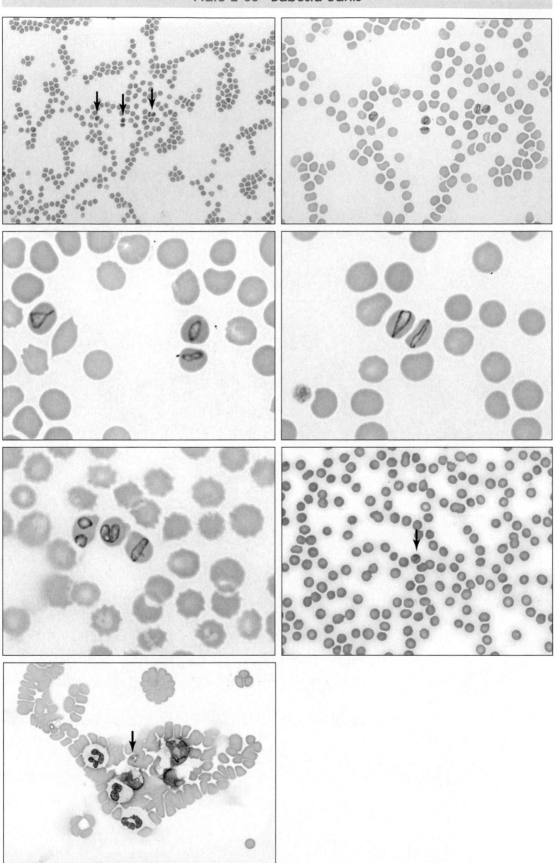

Make sure not to confuse Babesia organisms with **A,** Canine Distemper Inclusions **B,** Howell-Jolly bodies **C,** Basophilic stippling

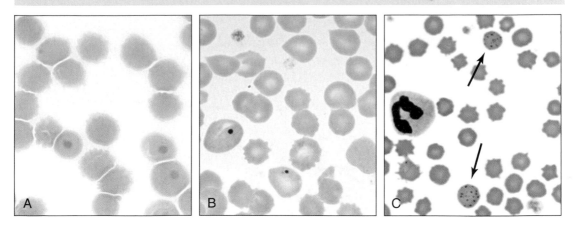

Plate 2-37 *Babesia gibsoni*

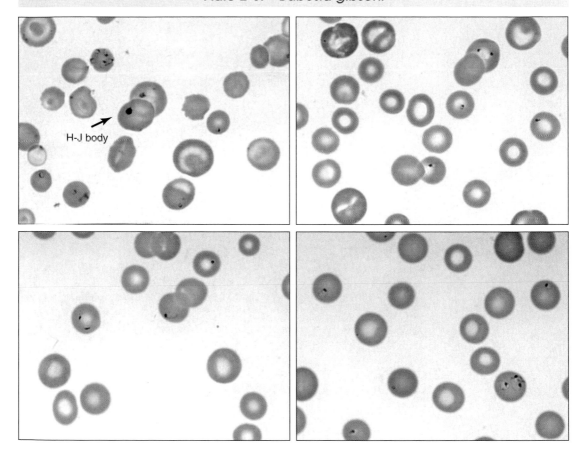

Plate 2-37 *Babesia gibsoni* (con't)

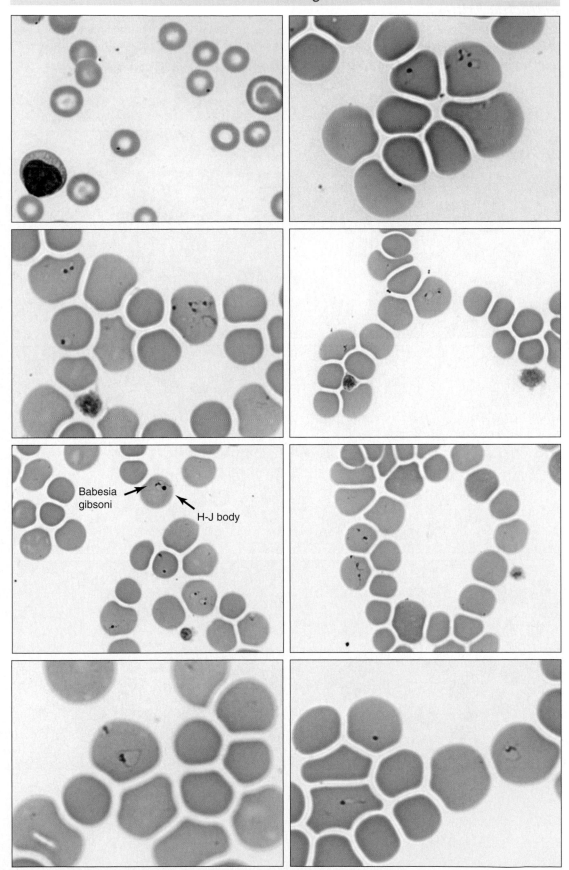

Babesia
gibsoni

H-J body

Red Blood Cell Artifacts

Refractile Artifact

DISTINCTIVE FEATURES: Refractile artifact is more commonly seen in Diff-Quik–stained smears as a slightly irregular, refractile clear spot seen on RBCs upon adjusting the fine focus of the microscope.

DIAGNOSTIC SIGNIFICANCE: Do not confuse refractile artifact with an RBC parasite or inclusion.

Plate 2-38   Refractile Artifact of Red Blood Cell

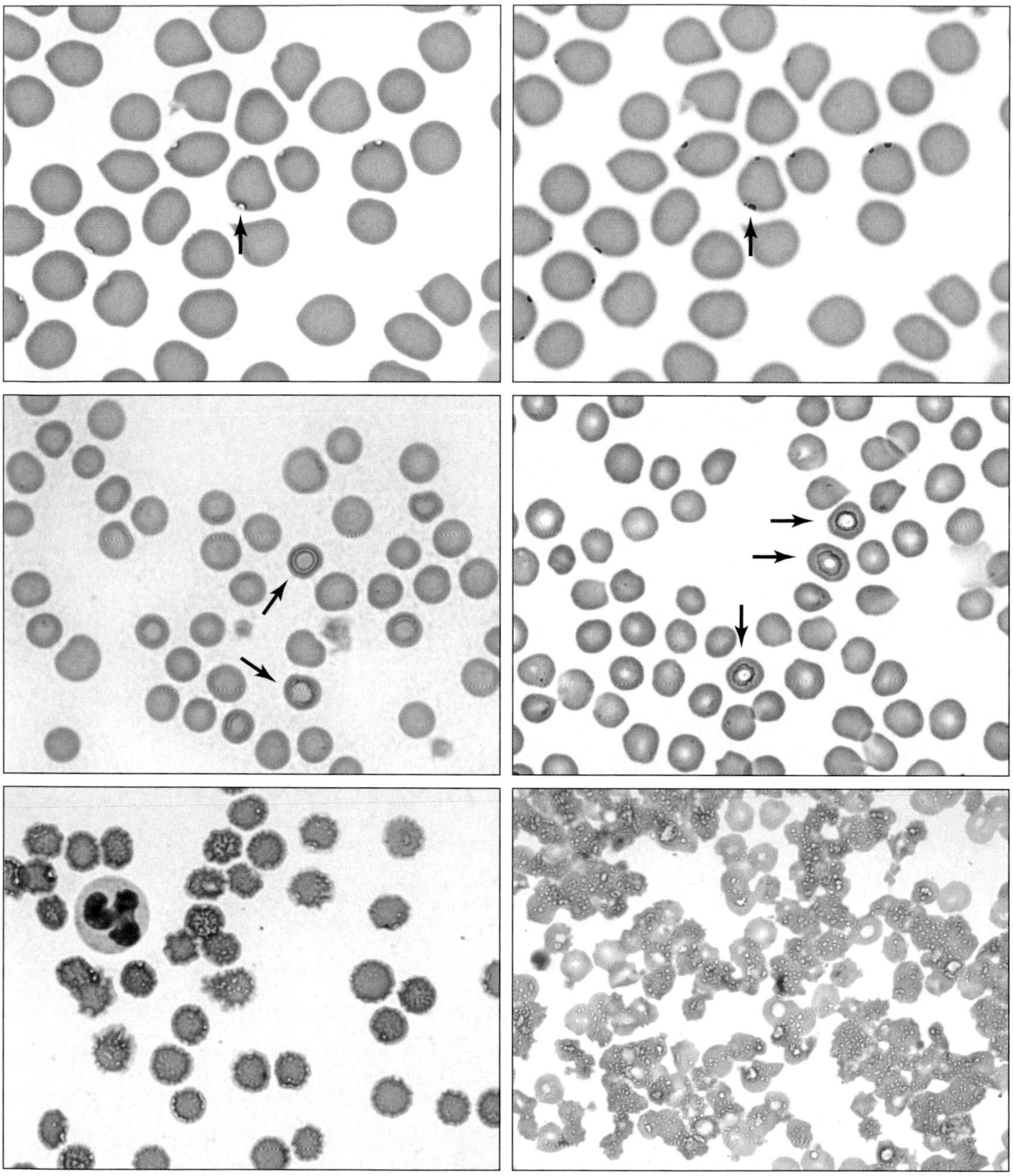

Plate 2-38 Refractile Artifact of Red Blood Cell *(con't)*

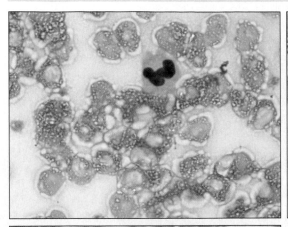
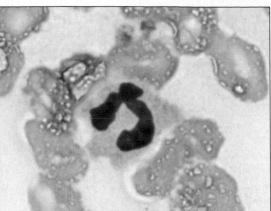
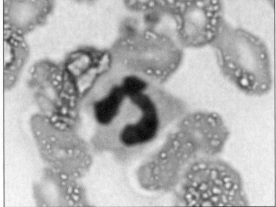

Platelet over Red Blood Cell

DISTINCTIVE FEATURES: Occasionally platelets will overlie RBCs and may be readily identified by adjusting the fine focus of the microscope and comparing the size and morphology to other platelets on the smear.

DIAGNOSTIC SIGNIFICANCE: Do not confuse platelets overlying RBCs with hemoparasites or inclusions.

Plate 2-39   Platelets Overlying Red Blood Cells

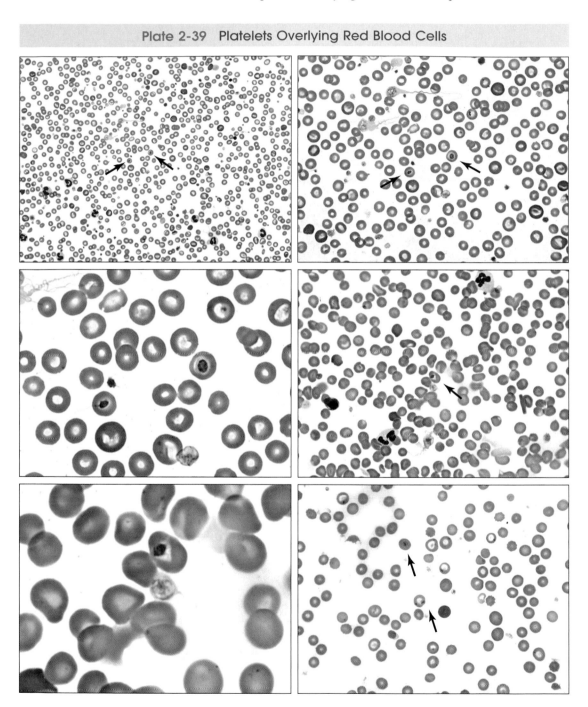

Plate 2-39 Platelets Overlying Red Blood Cells *(con't)*

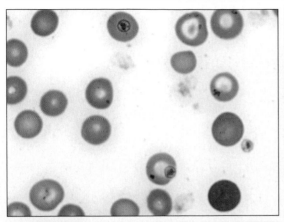

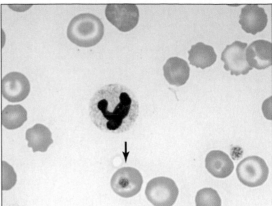

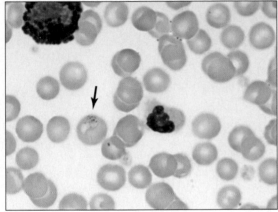

SECTION 3:
WHITE BLOOD CELLS

Normal Leukocyte Count

DIAGNOSTIC SIGNIFICANCE: A scan of the blood film may determine relative numbers of blood leukocytes and may be used to provide quality control of complete blood count (CBC) results obtained by hematology analyzers. The presence of normal numbers of leukocytes does not rule out disease of infectious, inflammatory, or neoplastic origin, emphasizing the need for careful microscopic review of cellular morphology.

Plate 3-1   Normal Leukocyte Count

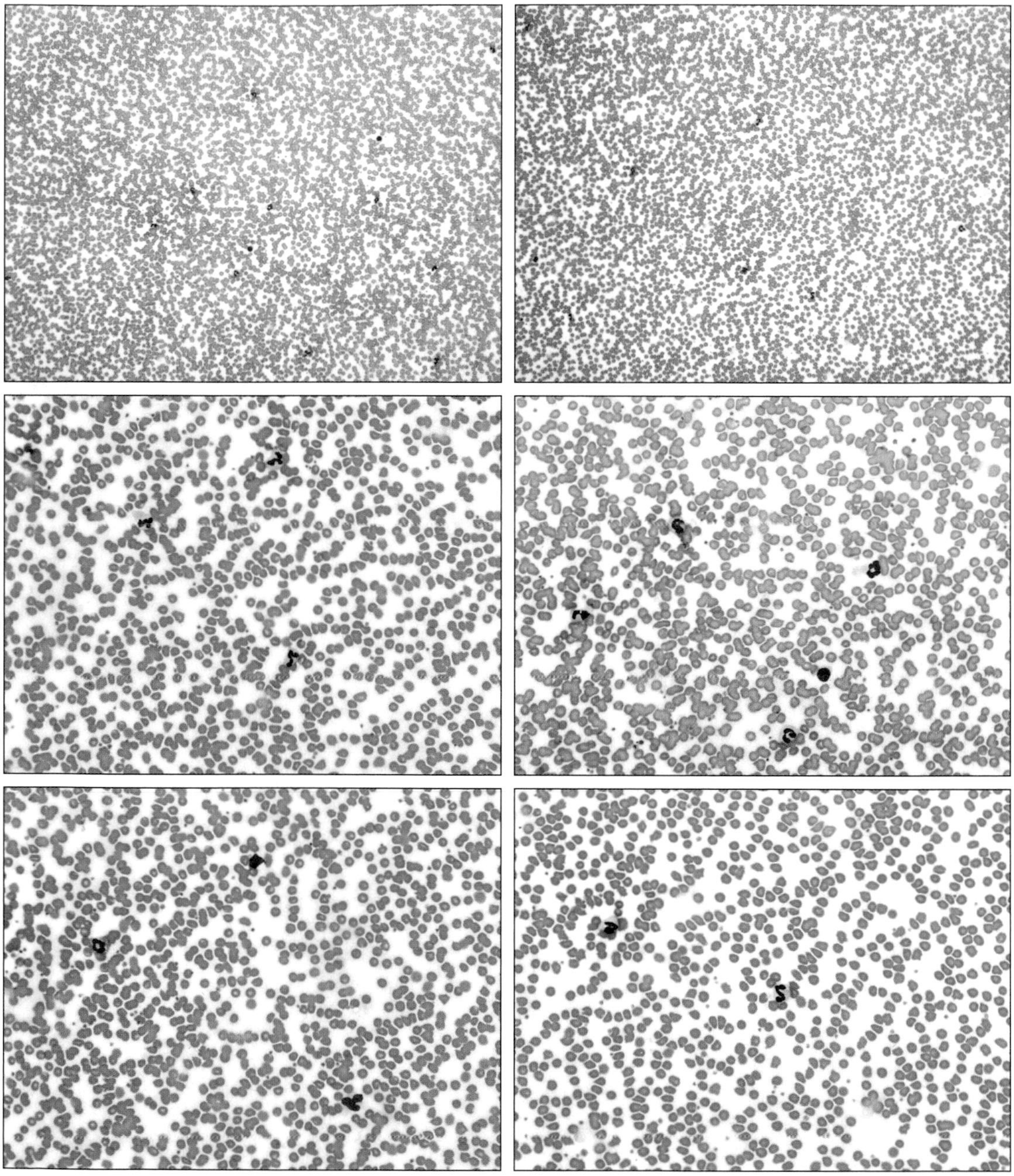

Plate 3-1 Normal Leukocyte Count *(con't)*

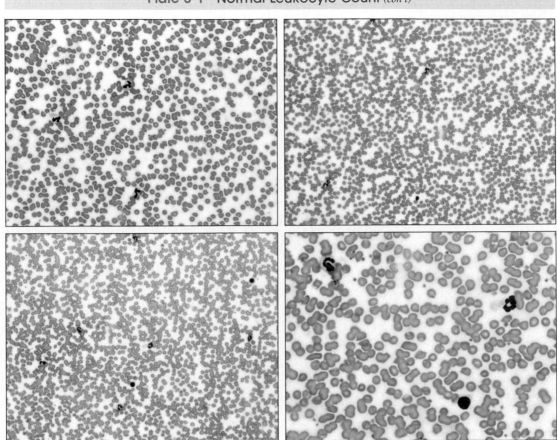

Leukocytosis

DIAGNOSTIC SIGNIFICANCE: Leukocytosis is defined as the presence of increased leukocyte numbers, which may be caused by an increase in the number of one cell type or a combination of cell types. The significance of a leukocytosis is based on the degree of elevation, the cell types constituting the increase, and the cellular morphology (normal, dysplastic, toxic, neoplastic). Increased numbers of neutrophils secondary to inflammation is the most common cause of a leukocytosis.

Plate 3-2 Leukocytosis

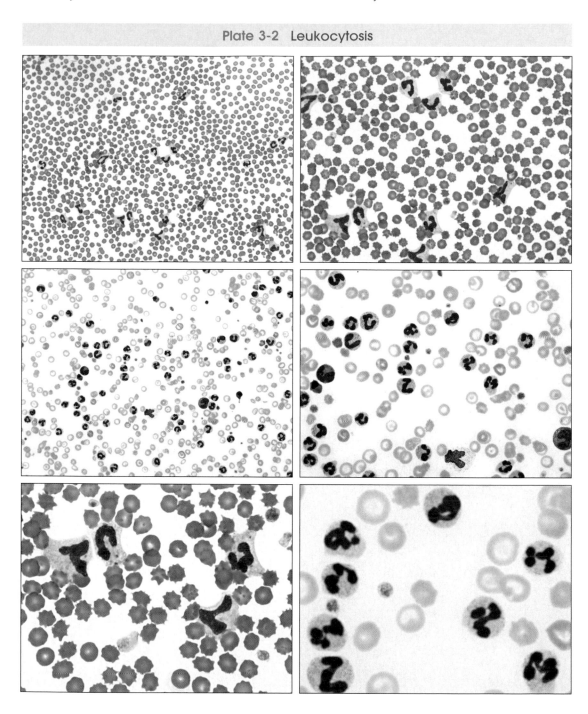

Plate 3-2 Leukocytosis *(con't)*

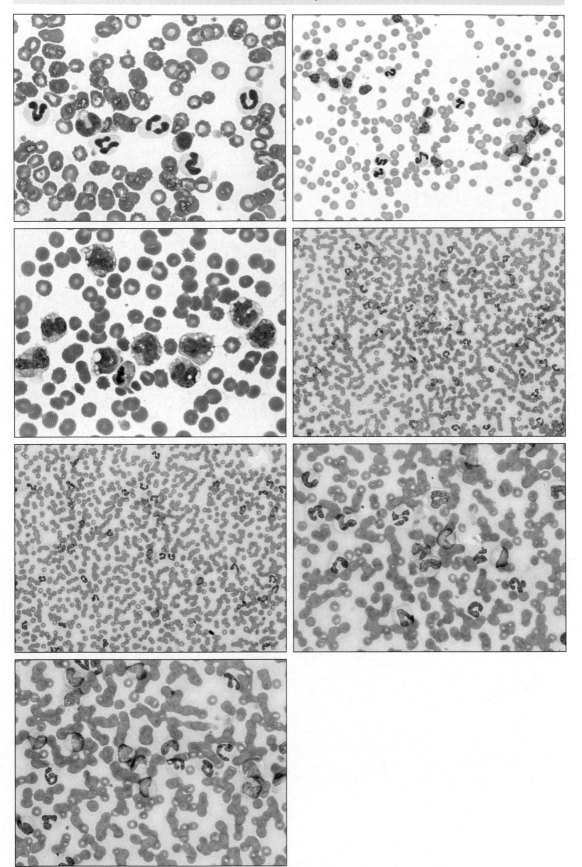

Leukopenia

DIAGNOSTIC SIGNIFICANCE: Leukopenia is defined as a decrease in leukocyte numbers, which is most often caused by a decrease in the number of neutrophils (neutropenia), as neutrophils are the most numerous of the peripheral blood leukocytes. Careful exam of the entire blood smear is emphasized by the fact that sometimes during blood smear preparation, the leukocytes can be concentrated on the feathered edge. In this case, the monolayer will contain very few leukocytes, suggesting an artifactual leukopenia if the monolayer only, and not the entire slide, is examined for WBC estimation.

Plate 3-3   Leukopenia

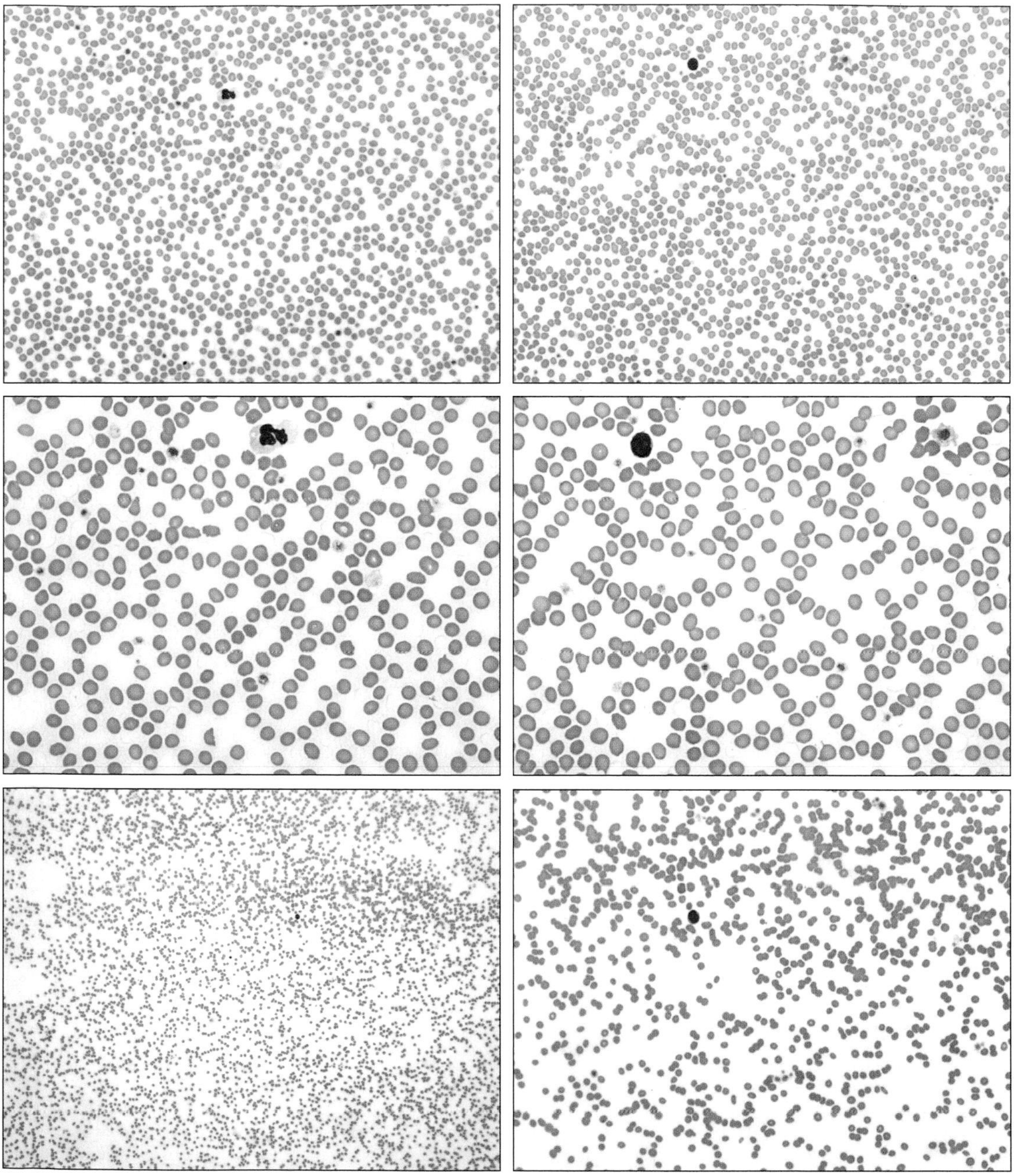

Plate 3-3 Leukopenia *(con't)*

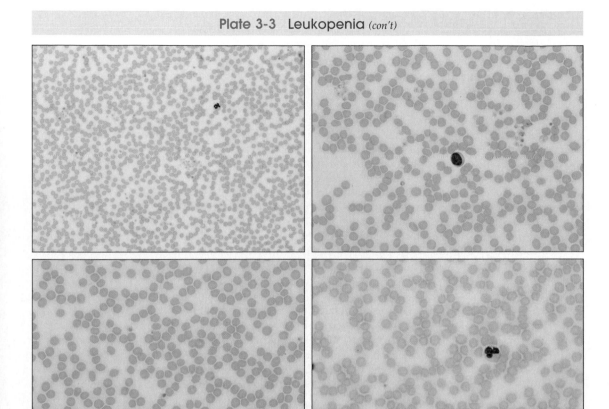

Artifactual leukopenia. **A,** Monolayer, devoid of leukocytes
B, Same smear where leukocytes are concentrated on the feathered edge

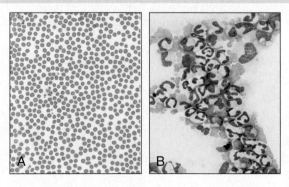

Neutrophils

Neutrophils are the most abundant of the granulocytic cell types. Maturation stages from least mature to most mature are: myeloblasts, promyelocytes, myelocytes, metamyelocytes, band neutrophils, and mature (segmented) neutrophils. As cells mature, they decrease in size, the cytoplasm becomes less blue and eventually becomes clear to lightly colored, and the nucleus becomes more condensed and eventually lobulated.

Neutrophils are released from bone marrow into circulation in an age-related fashion, with the most mature cells (mature neutrophils) released first. The bone marrow has a storage pool of mature neutrophils, so immature forms are not released into the circulation until the demand (severe, acute infection and inflammation) for neutrophils exceeds the storage pool's ability to supply adequate numbers of mature cells. Increased numbers of immature neutrophils in the peripheral blood is referred to as a "left shift" and is the hallmark of acute inflammation. Immature neutrophils are also released in an age-related fashion, and as such, the immature neutrophil stage primarily seen in peripheral blood during a left shift is the band neutrophil, with less mature stages seen only rarely. In general, the more severe the systemic inflammation, the higher the number of neutrophils with increased numbers of immature forms present.

The morphology and diagnostic significance of the various neutrophil maturational stages and the abnormalities that occur in the neutrophil series are discussed below.

Mature (Segmented) Neutrophils

DISTINCTIVE FEATURES: Mature neutrophils of dogs and cats have similar morphologies. Neutrophils are round and approximately 10 to 12 micrometers (μm) in diameter. The cytoplasm is clear, moderately abundant, and may contain a few very indistinct, faint pink granules, and/or small clear vacuoles, or both. The nucleus is highly condensed and lobulated, generally containing three or four lobules. Nuclear lobes may be connected by a thin strand of chromatin, but more commonly, simply a narrowing of the chromatin exists between lobes to about one third the diameter of the thick portion of the lobules.

DIAGNOSTIC SIGNIFICANCE: Mature neutrophil numbers are increased (neutrophilia) in conditions such as epinephrine release (from excitement), endogenous steroids (stress resulting in glucocorticoid release), steroid administration, inflammation (infectious and noninfectious causes), tissue necrosis, and neoplasia. Mature neutrophilia caused by inflammation is often associated with an increase in band neutrophils (left shift). *Leukemoid response* is a term used to describe a marked neutrophilia, often with a left shift, which may be seen with severe, acute, focal inflammation (i.e., pyometra, peritonitis, pyothorax, severe abscessation). A persistently increasing, moderate to marked neutrophilia, in which a source of inflammation, infection, tissue destruction, or necrosis cannot be found, should raise the suspicion for chronic granulocytic leukemia.

Mature neutrophil numbers are decreased (neutropenia) by conditions such as overwhelming bacterial infections, viral infections (parvovirus, panleukopenia, feline leukemia virus [FeLV]), certain bacterial infections (*Salmonella*), rickettsial infections (i.e., chronic ehrlichiosis), endotoxemia (infection with gram-negative bacteria), chemotherapeutic agents, bone marrow necrosis, myelophthesic diseases (bone marrow infiltration with neoplastic cells), and bone marrow suppression or failure (i.e., drug-induced neutropenia, immune-mediated neutropenia, cyclic hematopoiesis).

Plate 3-4 Normal Mature Segmented Neutrophils

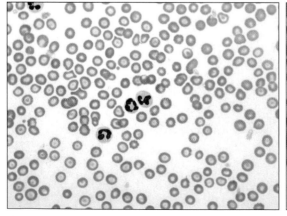 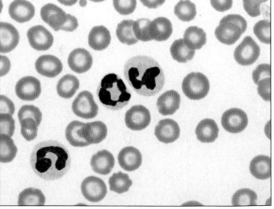

Plate 3-4 Normal Mature Segmented Neutrophils *(con't)*

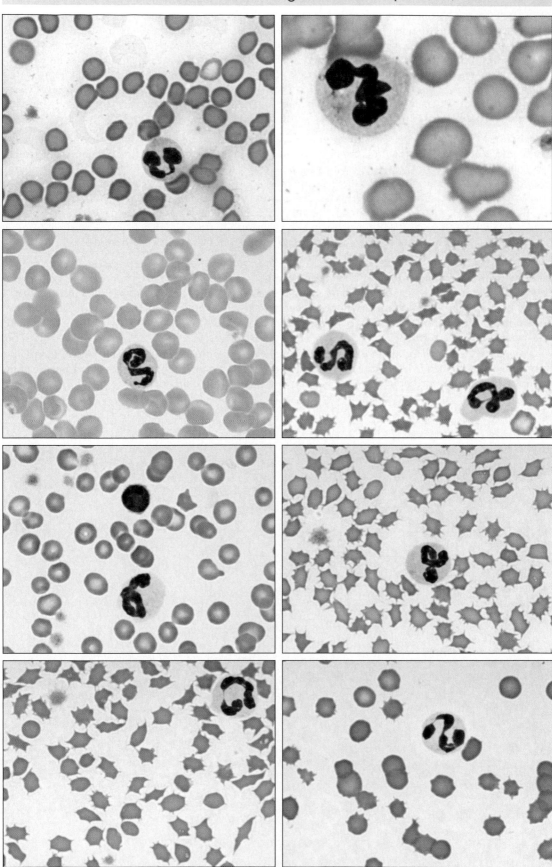

Band Neutrophils

DISTINCTIVE FEATURES: Band neutrophils are similar in size and appearance to mature neutrophils except that the nuclei are nonsegmented (band shaped) or only slightly constricted, and nuclear chromatin is not as tightly clumped. The classic band neutrophil has a plump C-shaped or S-shaped nucleus, with parallel sides, a smooth nuclear margin, and a fairly constant width. If slight constricted areas are present, they are more than one third the width of the rest of the nucleus, distinguishing the bands from mature neutrophils, which have constricted areas of less than one third the width of other areas of the nucleus. The nuclear chromatin is less dense than that of a mature neutrophil. The cytoplasm remains clear unless toxic change is present.

DIAGNOSTIC SIGNIFICANCE: Band neutrophils are either absent or present in very low numbers in healthy dogs and cats. A left shift is the hallmark of acute inflammation. Systemic inflammatory mediators travel to bone marrow, resulting in the production and release of neutrophils. Despite this systemic response, the inflammation may be focal (i.e., pyometra) or diffuse (i.e., bacterial sepsis). Additionally, not all focal areas of inflammation induce a systemic response. For example, cystitis (inflammation of the bladder) is not generally associated with an increased number of band neutrophils. Chronic granulocytic leukemia may also cause an increase in band neutrophil numbers. Also, pseudo–band neutrophils (hyposegmented mature neutrophils) may be seen in Pelger-Huët anomaly (discussed later).

A left shift may be regenerative or degenerative. A regenerative left shift is a predominance of mature neutrophils (neutrophilia) with fewer bands, indicating a normal response to inflammation. A degenerative left shift occurs when bands (and often more immature forms of neutrophils) exceed the number of mature neutrophils. Often, a concurrent neutropenia exists. This indicates neutrophil production is not able to meet demand and is associated with a guarded or poor prognosis. Toxic changes are frequent with degenerative left shifts.

As band neutrophils are the most common immature neutrophil released into peripheral blood and cannot be distinguished from mature neutrophils with current hematology analyzers, blood smear evaluation is extremely important in identifying and quantitating a left shift.

Plate 3-5   Band Neutrophils

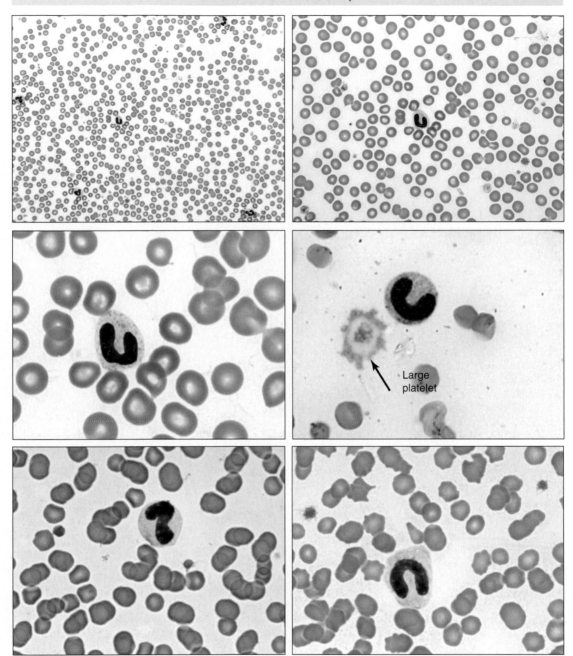

Large
platelet

Plate 3-5 Band Neutrophils *(con't)*

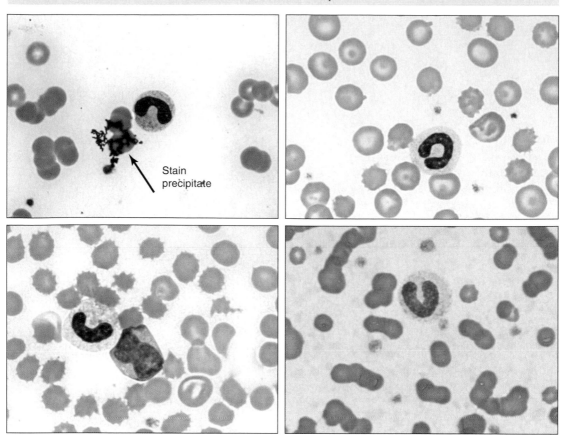

Stain
precipitate

A, Band neutrophils. Note the open chromatin
B, Neutrophils with Pelger-Huët Anomaly. Note the condensed chromatin

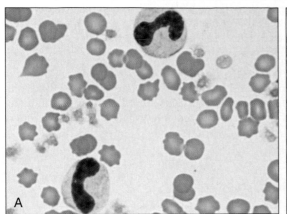
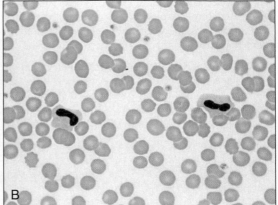

Metamyelocytes

DISTINCTIVE FEATURES: Metamyelocytes are about the same size to slightly larger than mature and band neutrophils. The nuclei have one margin indented more than 25% into the nucleus and have an indented or kidney-shaped nucleus. The nuclear chromatin is readily recognized as condensed but generally less so than that of band neutrophils. The cytoplasm is nearly colorless but more basophilic than the nontoxic band neutrophil.

DIAGNOSTIC SIGNIFICANCE: Metamyelocytes are rarely seen in the peripheral blood of healthy dogs and cats. Metamyelocytes are sometimes seen in peripheral blood during severe inflammation along with band neutrophils as part of a left shift. Granulocytic leukemia may also cause an increase in metamyelocytes but occurs rarely. Also, pseudometamyelocytes (hyposegmented mature neutrophils) may be seen in Pelger-Huët anomaly (discussed later).

Plate 3-6   Metamyelocytes

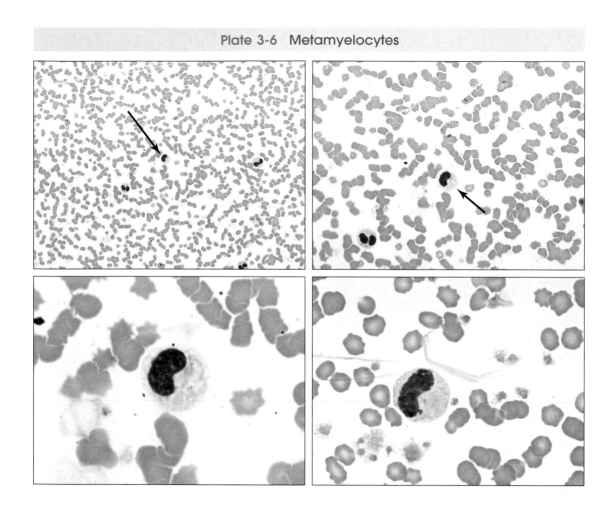

Plate 3-6 Metamyelocytes (con't)

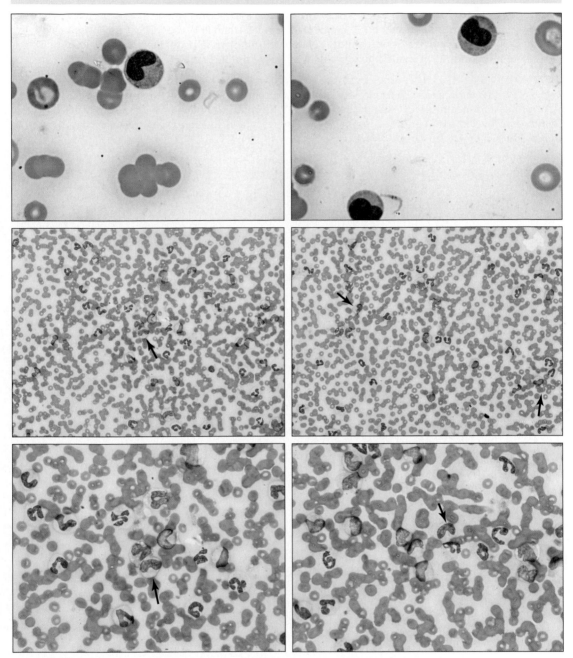

Myelocytes

DISTINCTIVE FEATURES: Myelocytes are about the same size to slightly larger than metamyelocytes. The nuclei are often slightly indented, but the indentation is less than 25% the thickness of the nucleus. The chromatin of metamyelocytes is only mildly condensed and often appears more open. The cytoplasm is clear, pale blue, and may contain a few visible magenta-staining granules.

DIAGNOSTIC SIGNIFICANCE: Myelocytes are rarely seen in the peripheral blood of healthy dogs and cats. A few myelocytes may be found in peripheral blood during severe inflammation along with band neutrophils and metamyelocytes as part of a left shift. Chronic granulocytic leukemia may also cause an increase in myelocytes. Also, pseudomyelocytes (hyposegmented mature neutrophils) may be seen in Pelger-Huët anomaly (discussed later).

Plate 3-7 Myelocytes

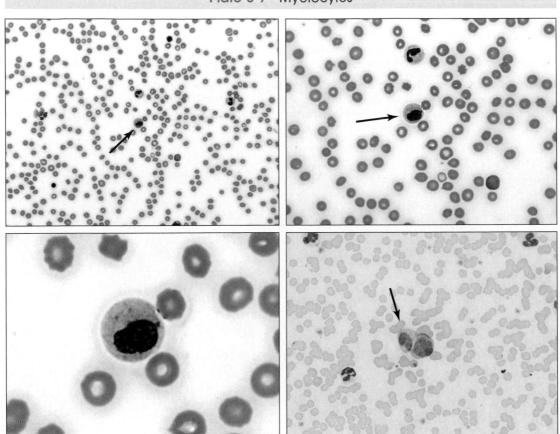

Promyelocytes

DISTINCTIVE FEATURES: Promyelocytes are slightly larger than myelocytes. The nuclei are round to oval, with lacy to coarse chromatin without distinct clumps of condensed chromatin. Nuclei of a few promyelocytes may contain visible nucleoli or nuclear rings, but most do not. The cytoplasm is light blue and contains numerous magenta-staining granules, the latter being a hallmark feature of promyelocytes.

DIAGNOSTIC SIGNIFICANCE: Promyelocytes are rarely seen in the peripheral blood of healthy dogs and cats. A few promyelocytes may occasionally be seen in peripheral blood during severe inflammation along with bands, metamyelocytes, and myelocytes as part of a left shift. Chronic granulocytic leukemia may also cause an increase in promyelocytes.

Plate 3-8   Promyelocytes

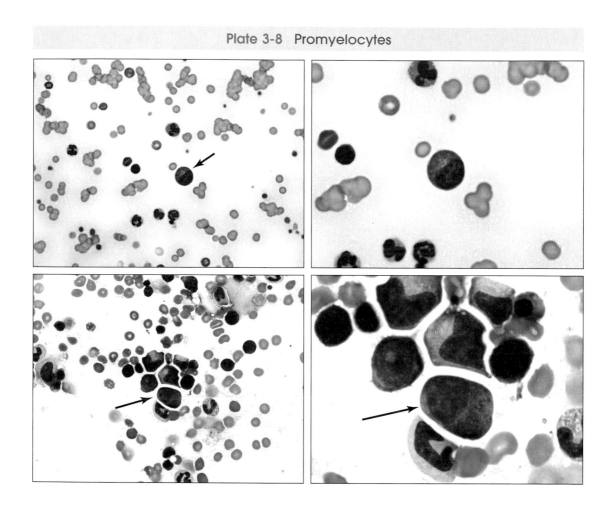

Plate 3-8 Promyelocytes *(con't)*

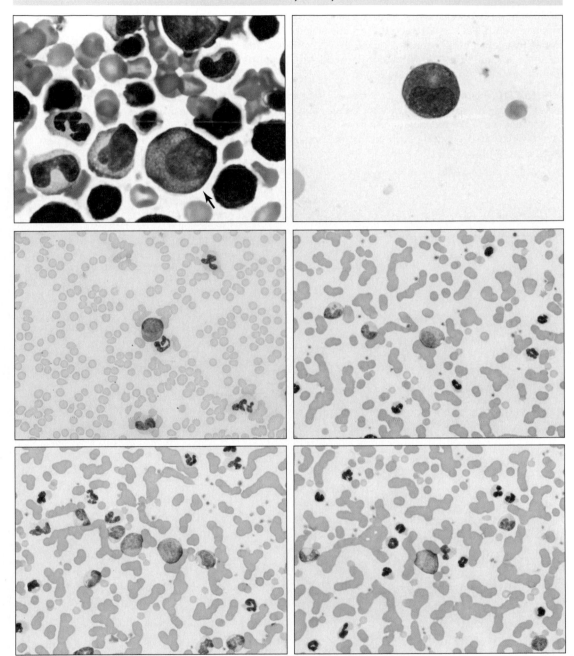

Myeloblasts

DISTINCTIVE FEATURES: Myeloblasts are difficult to distinguish from the primitive blasts of other hematopoietic cell lines. They are about the same size as, or slightly smaller than, promyelocytes. They have round to oval, centrally located nuclei that have finely stippled chromatin and one to several visible nucleoli. A small to moderate amount of moderately basophilic cytoplasm may contain a few fine azurophilic granules (primary granules).

DIAGNOSTIC SIGNIFICANCE: It is extremely rare to see myeloblasts in the peripheral blood smears of healthy dogs and cats. Finding a myeloblast on a peripheral blood smear always raises the possibility of granulocytic leukemia; however, a myeloblast may rarely be seen on a peripheral blood smear during severe inflammation, along with bands, metamyelocytes, myelocytes, and promyelocytes as part of a left shift.

Plate 3-9 Myeloblasts

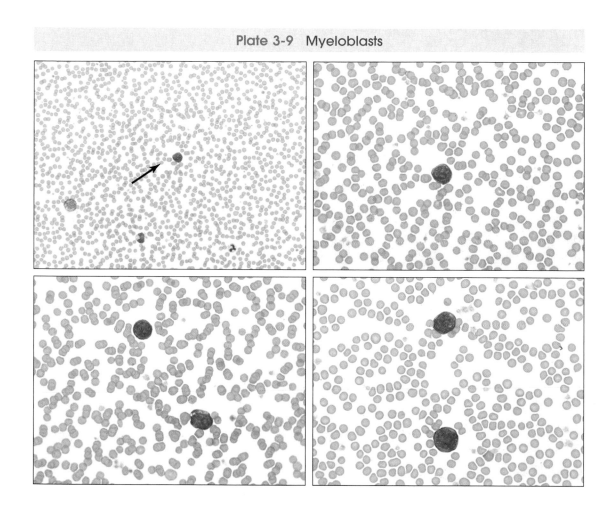

Plate 3-9 Myeloblasts *(con't)*

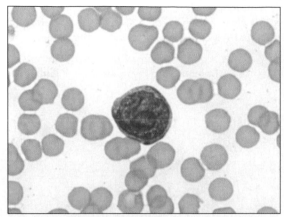

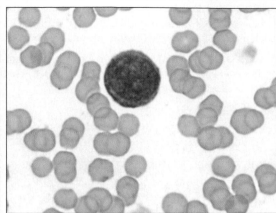

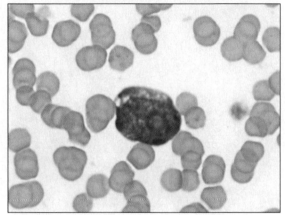

Barr Body

DISTINCTIVE FEATURES: The nucleus of some neutrophils of females may have a single visible Barr body. A Barr body is a small, well-defined, "drumsticklike" nuclear appendage attached to the neutrophil nucleus by a slender chromatin strand. Barr bodies are usually located near one end of the nucleus.

DIAGNOSTIC SIGNIFICANCE: Barr bodies represent the inactive X chromosome of the female. Rare Barr body–like projections may be seen in males because of chance segmentation in the neutrophil. Barr bodies have no diagnostic significance.

Plate 3-10   Barr Bodies

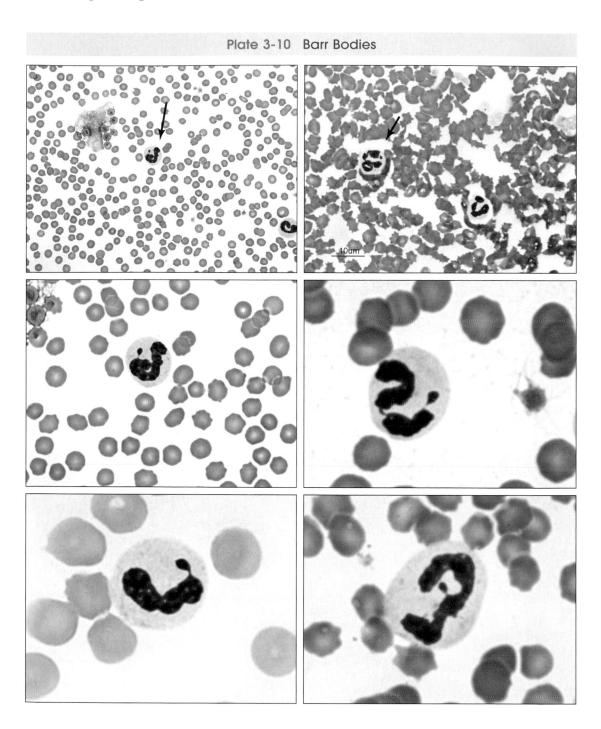

Plate 3-10 Barr Bodies (con't)

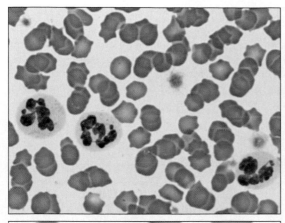

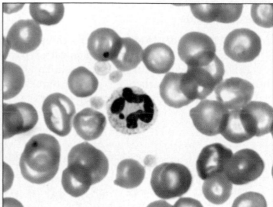

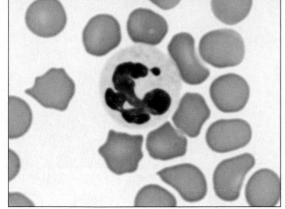

Hypersegmented Neutrophils

DISTINCTIVE FEATURES: Neutrophils with five or more distinct nuclear lobes are classified as hypersegmented.

DIAGNOSTIC SIGNIFICANCE: Hypersegmentation is an aging change, which may occur as an in vitro artifact secondary to delayed blood smear preparation (several hours) from ethylenediaminetetraacetic acid (EDTA)–anticoagulated blood; a cellular aging change caused by prolonged blood transit time (i.e., chronic excess glucocorticoids), as an acquired defect (i.e., B_{12} or folic acid deficiency, FeLV myelodysplasia), or as an inherited maturation defect (i.e., macrocytosis of poodles).

Plate 3-11   Hypersegmented Neutrophils

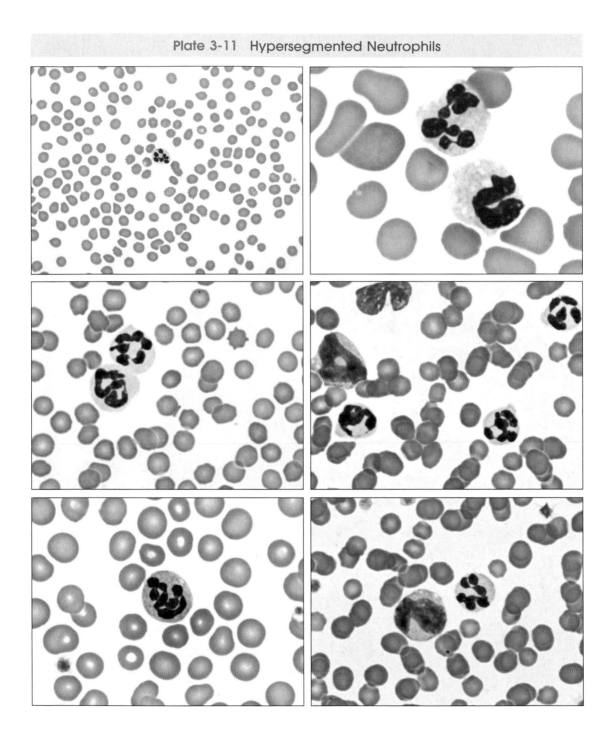

Plate 3-11   Hypersegmented Neutrophils *(con't)*

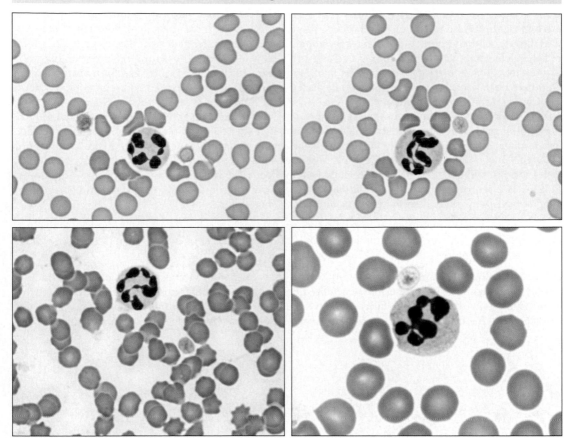

Pelger-Huët and Pseudo-Pelger-Huët Neutrophils

DISTINCTIVE FEATURES: Pelger-Huët and pseudo-Pelger-Huët neutrophils are mature neutrophils that are hyposegmented because of an inherited (Pelger-Huët) or acquired (pseudo–Pelger-Huët) defect in granulocyte segmentation, which creates the appearance of a persistent left shift. The heterozygous form of Pelger-Huët anomaly is seen in dogs and cats and is clinically benign as neutrophils function normally. The homozygous state in utero is generally fatal. Hyposegmentation is recognized by the mature (coarsely clumped) nuclear chromatin in relation to the lack of segmentation of the cell. Hyposegmentation occurs in other peripheral blood leukocytes (i.e., eosinophils) but is most easily recognized in neutrophils because of their predominant number and normally segmented nuclei. Nuclei of mature Pelger-Huet neutrophils may be round, oval, band-shaped, dumb-bell shaped, or bilobed. Lack of toxic change and lack of illness or clinical signs in what appears to be a marked left shift are important in the identification of Pelger-Huët anomaly. Pelger-Huët neutrophils are easily recognized if the animal is not sick; however, if the animal is ill and Pelger-Huët anomaly has not been previously documented, then recognition of Pelger-Huët neutrophils may be very difficult. If the patient becomes well following treatment, and the left shift fails to resolve, then Pelger-Huët anomaly is most likely.

With resolving chronic inflammatory disease, an acquired pseudo-Pelger-Huët disorder is likely to occur. This is very rare and is differentiated from true Pelger-Huët anomaly, as the nuclear hyposegmentation resolves together with the inflammation.

DIAGNOSTIC SIGNIFICANCE: Careful morphologic assessment of cytoplasmic and nuclear features is important in distinguishing inherited or acquired Pelger-Huët anomaly from a true left shift. Correlation of the findings with the health status of the patient is very important. If the patient is sick, continued assessment of the blood film over time may be necessary to rule out Pelger-Huët anomaly.

Plate 3-12 Pelger-Huët Anomaly

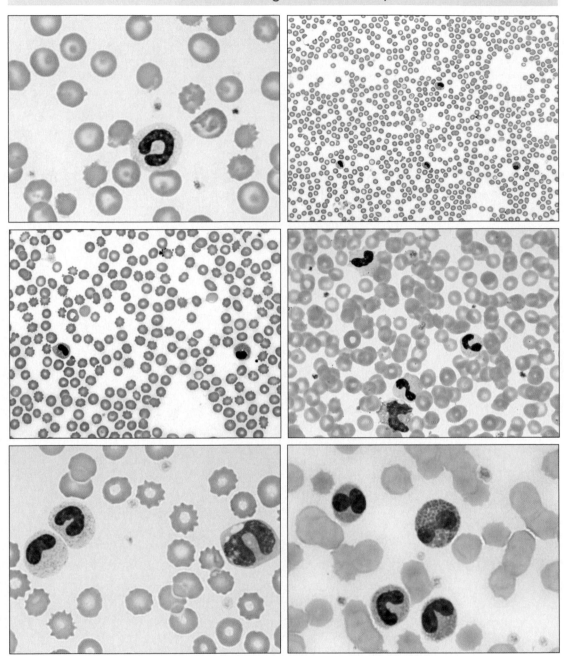

Plate 3-12   Pelger-Huët Anomaly *(con't)*

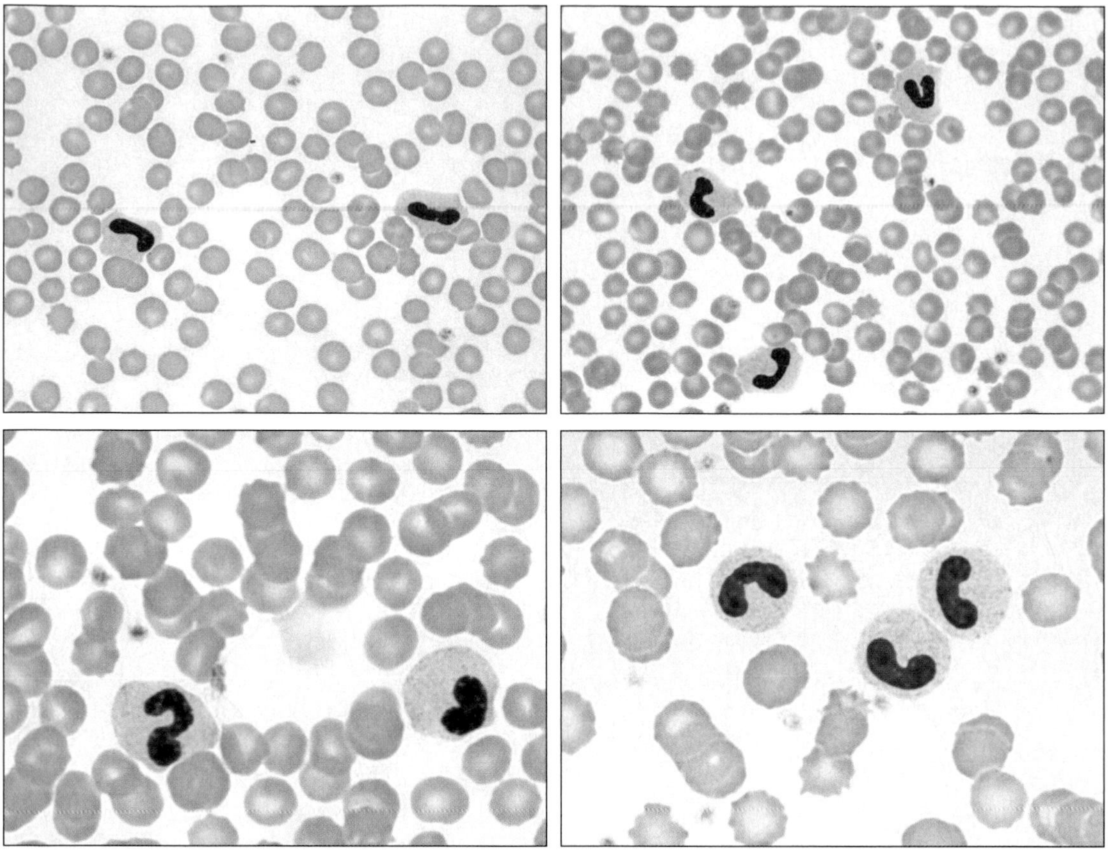

A, Band neutrophils. Note the open chromatin
B, Neutrophils seen with Pelger-Huët Anomaly. Note the condensed chromatin

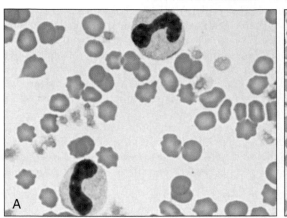

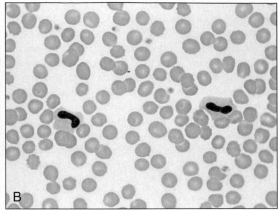

Toxic Changes

Systemic inflammation, most notably secondary to bacterial infections, may cause microscopic toxic changes in neutrophils. The most common toxic changes are cytoplasmic and include Döhle bodies, toxic granulation, diffuse cytoplasmic basophilia, and cytoplasmic vacuolation. Toxic neutrophils may contain only one or two of these changes, or all may be evident in severely toxic cells. During rapid neutrophil production (neutropoiesis) in bone marrow in response to systemic inflammatory mediators, neutrophils undergo specific maturation defects, which results in toxic changes. As with a left shift, the presence of toxic neutrophils indicates systemic inflammation. Less common toxic changes involve the nucleus (i.e., ring forms) or affect cell size (i.e., giant neutrophils) and are rarely seen except with severe inflammation, often with a significant left shift.

Like band neutrophils and other immature neutrophil forms, toxic neutrophils are not recognized by automated hematology analyzers and must be identified on blood film review. The different toxic changes discussed below are generally graded as slight, mild, moderate, or marked; or on a 1 to 4+ scale. In general, the more pronounced the toxic change and the higher the percentage of toxic neutrophils, the higher is the grade.

Döhle Bodies

DISTINCTIVE FEATURES: Döhle bodies are variably sized, variably shaped, light blue to slate gray structures in the cytoplasm of neutrophils. These foci are clumps of endoplasmic reticulum that are usually degraded during maturation, yet retained during accelerated neutropoiesis.

DIAGNOSTIC SIGNIFICANCE: Döhle bodies are the most easily produced and, therefore, the most common form of toxic change observed in neutrophils. Regardless of the number of neutrophils containing Döhle bodies, when occurring alone without other toxic changes, Döhle bodies should never be interpreted as meaning anything more than a mild toxic change in dogs. Döhle bodies may occur in clinically healthy cats and, thus, are often not reported as a toxic change in cats unless these bodies are numerous or present with other toxic changes. Make sure not to confuse Döhle with *Ehrlichia* morulae and Distemper inclusions or platelets overlying WBCs.

NEXT STEPS: When Döhle bodies are evident in the dog or seen in high numbers in cats, assess for other toxic changes and for the presence of immature neutrophils (left shift). Be careful to not confuse Döhle bodies with *Ehrlichia* morulae, distemper inclusions, or parasites.

Plate 3-13 Döhle Bodies

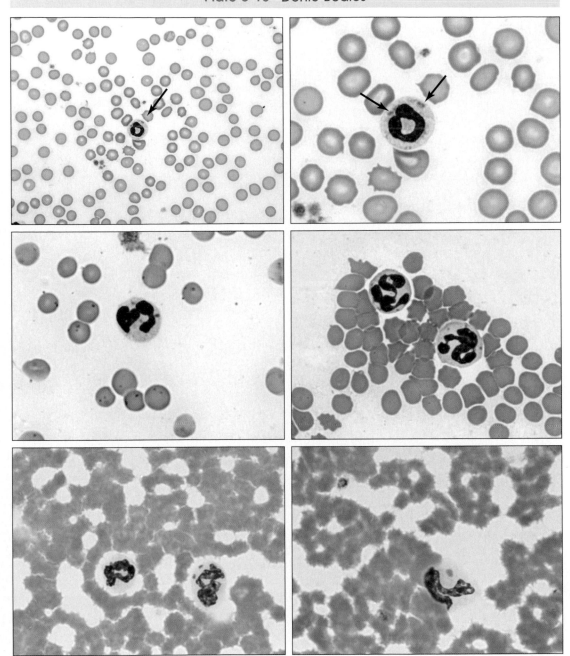

Plate 3-13   Döhle Bodies *(con't)*

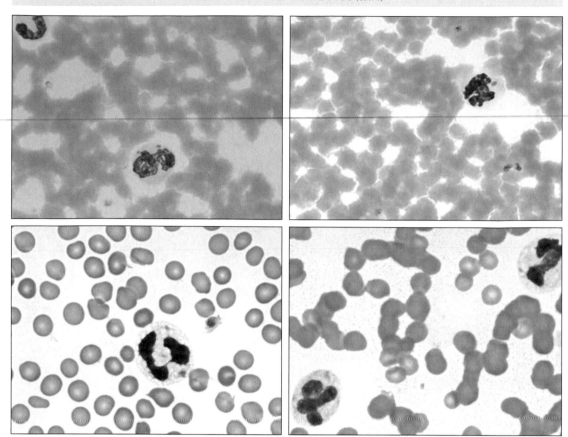

A, Döhle bodies **B,** Canine neutrophil with *Ehrlichia* morulae
C, Distemper inclusions **D,** Platelet over neutrophil

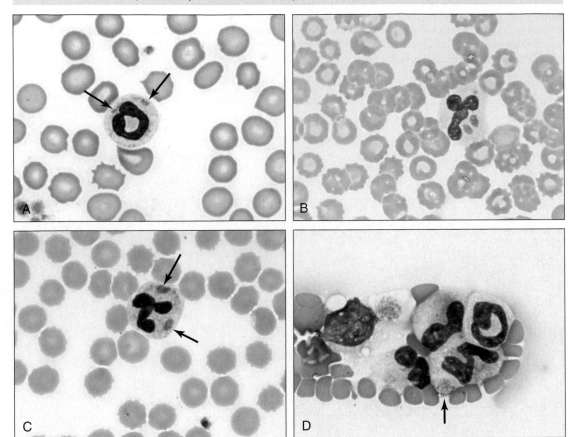

Diffuse Cytoplasmic Basophilia

DISTINCTIVE FEATURES: With diffuse cytoplasmic basophilia, the neutrophil cytoplasm stains basophilic (blue). Diffuse basophilia occurs when ribosomes remain scattered throughout the cytoplasm (as opposed to being clumped into Döhle bodies), instead of being degraded during maturation. Diffuse cytoplasmic basophilia is graded as a mild, moderate, or severe, depending on the number of neutrophils affected and the severity of the basophilia.

DIAGNOSTIC SIGNIFICANCE: The presence of diffuse cytoplasmic basophilia indicates systemic inflammation, regardless of whether a neutrophilia or a left shift exists (although it usually is associated with both).

Plate 3-14 Cytoplasmic Basophilia

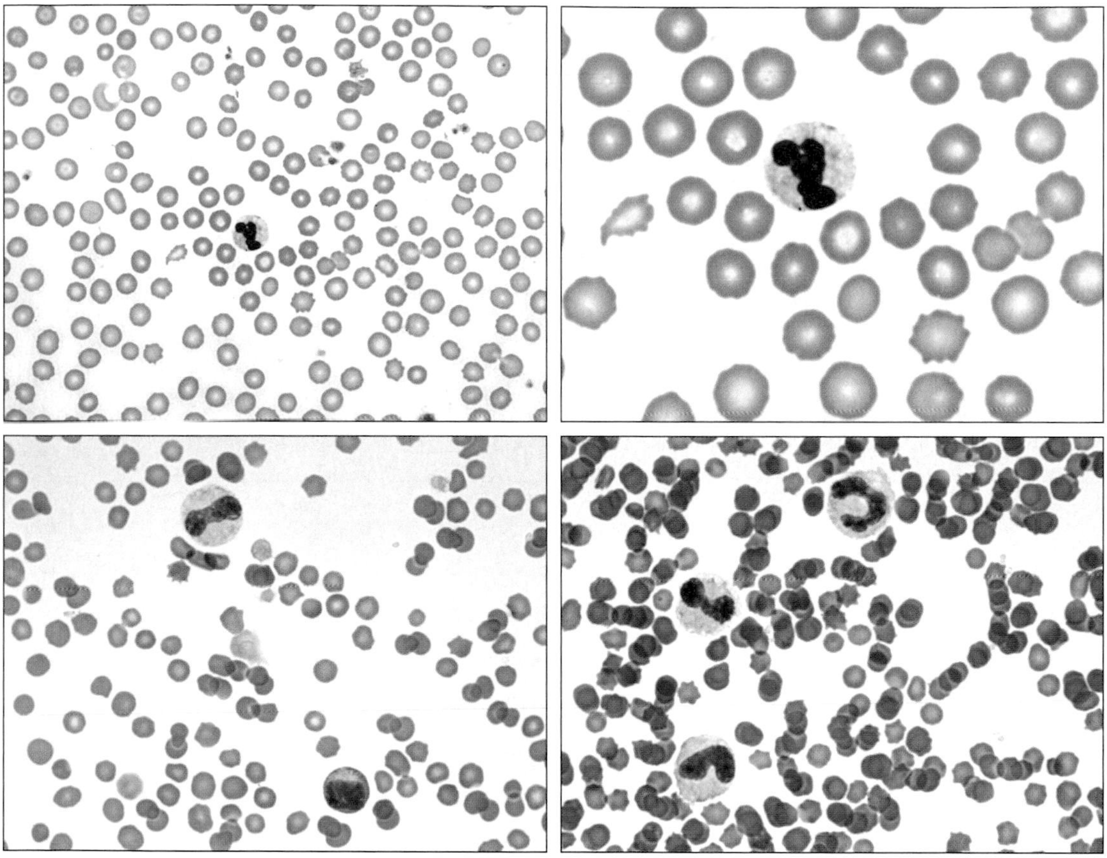

Plate 3-14 Cytoplasmic Basophilia *(con't)*

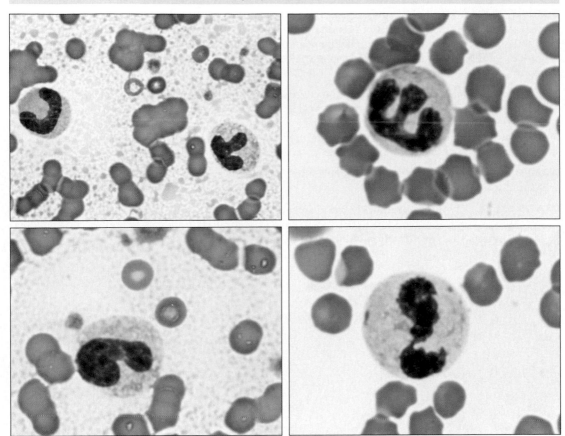

Cytoplasmic Vacuolization (Foamy Cytoplasm)

DISTINCTIVE FEATURES: Neutrophils containing foamy appearing vacuoles within their cytoplasm are considered toxic. Toxic vacuolization generally is recognized in association with diffuse cytoplasmic basophilia, as the basophilic background enhances the ability to discern the vacuoles. Toxic vacuolization is graded as mild, moderate, or severe, depending on the number of neutrophils affected and the degree of vacuolization.

Cytoplasmic vacuolization should not be confused with the discrete clear vacuoles that develop in neutrophils exposed to EDTA for several hours. The rate of EDTA-induced cytoplasmic vacuolization is variable, depending on temperature and other factors, but may occur rather rapidly. Therefore, if cytoplasmic vacuolization is present without other evidence of inflammation (i.e., other toxic changes, left shift), the possibility of artifactual cytoplasmic vacuolization should be considered.

DIAGNOSTIC SIGNIFICANCE: Toxic vacuolization occurs secondary to systemic inflammation or artifactually.

NEXT STEPS: Determine how quickly blood smears were made from the EDTA blood tube. Prolonged exposure of peripheral blood to EDTA before smear preparation is the most common cause of artifactual cytoplasmic vacuolization within neutrophils.

Plate 3-15 Cytoplasmic Vacuolization

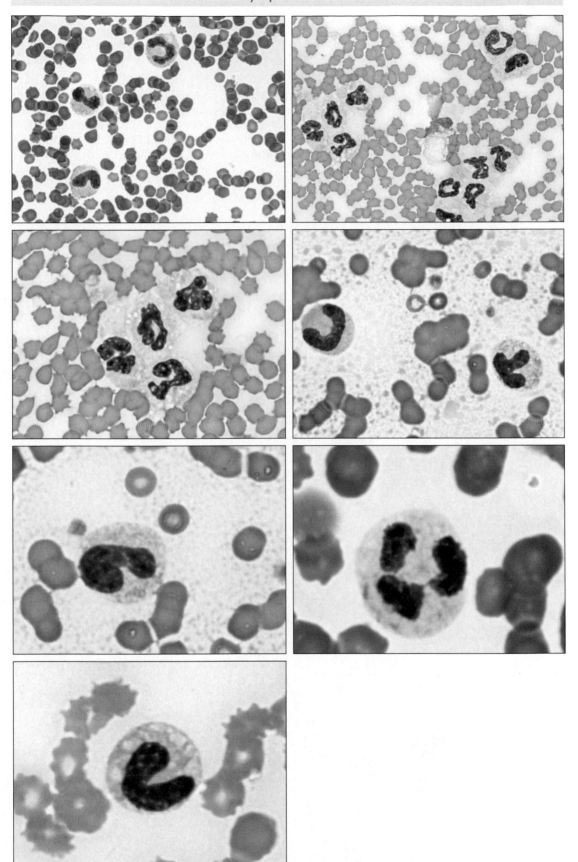

Toxic Granulation

DISTINCTIVE FEATURES: Neutrophils containing low to high numbers of magenta-staining cytoplasmic granules are toxic. These are retained primary granules, which are not normally present in later stages of neutrophil development (usually seen up to the progranulocyte stage). Depending on the number of neutrophils affected, toxic granulation is interpreted as a mild, moderate, or severe.

DIAGNOSTIC SIGNIFICANCE Toxic granulation indicates systemic inflammation.

NEXT STEPS: If neutrophilic granulation is observed without evidence of other toxic changes, a left shift, or both, and a source of inflammation or infection is not evident, consider uncommon hereditary diseases associated with neutrophil inclusions, for example, Chédiak-Higashi syndrome in blue-smoke Persian cats (usually abnormal granules are also seen in eosinophils and basophils); GM$_2$ gangliosidosis (German Shorthaired Pointers and some cats [dark blue granules are seen in neutrophils and azurophilic granules in lymphocytes]); Birman cat anomaly (seen in purebred Birman cats); mucopolysaccharidosis (MPS) type VI (Siamese and Domestic Shorthair cats and Dachshunds); and MPS type VII (neutrophilic inclusions are seen in dogs and cats with this disorder).

Plate 3-16 Toxic Granulation

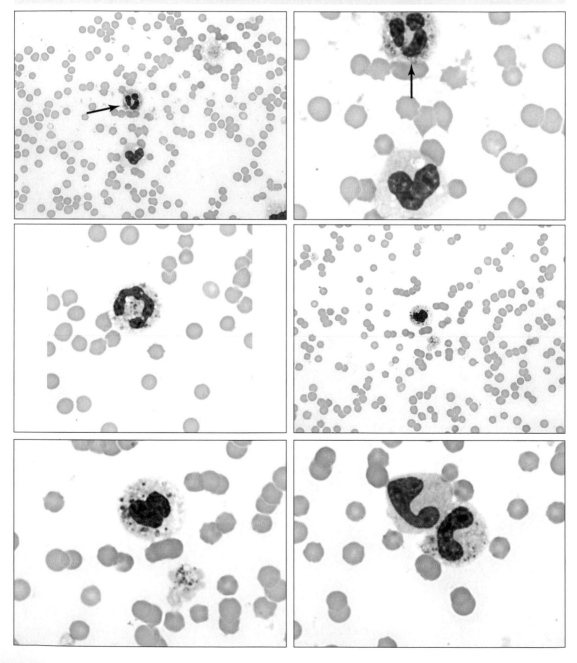

Plate 3-16 Toxic Granulation *(con't)*

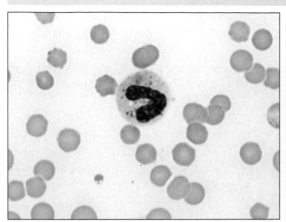

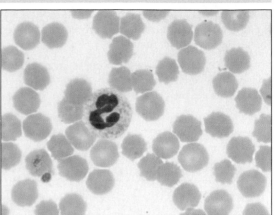

A, Toxic granulation **B,** Mucopolysaccharidosis **C,** Birman Cat Anomaly
D, Chédiak-Higashi Syndrome **E,** Primary neutrophil granules

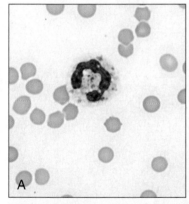

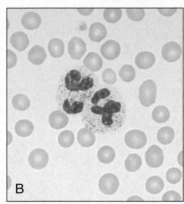

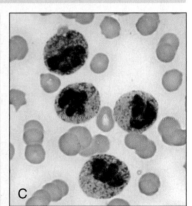

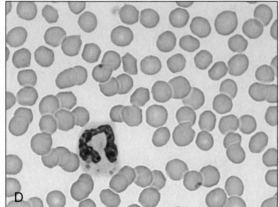

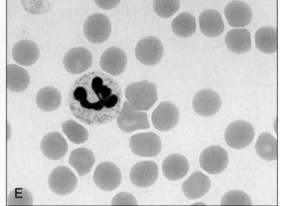

Ring (Doughnut) Form

DISTINCTIVE FEATURES: Immature neutrophils containing a round nucleus with a hole in the center (doughnut-shaped nucleus) without significant indentations in the nucleus are a rarely observed toxic change involving the nucleus.

DIAGNOSTIC SIGNIFICANCE: Ring-form neutrophils are seen occasionally in cats and infrequently in dogs with severe systemic inflammation or toxemia. This finding is considered a toxic change, and the neutrophils are best classified as band neutrophils.

Plate 3-17   Ring-Form Neutrophils

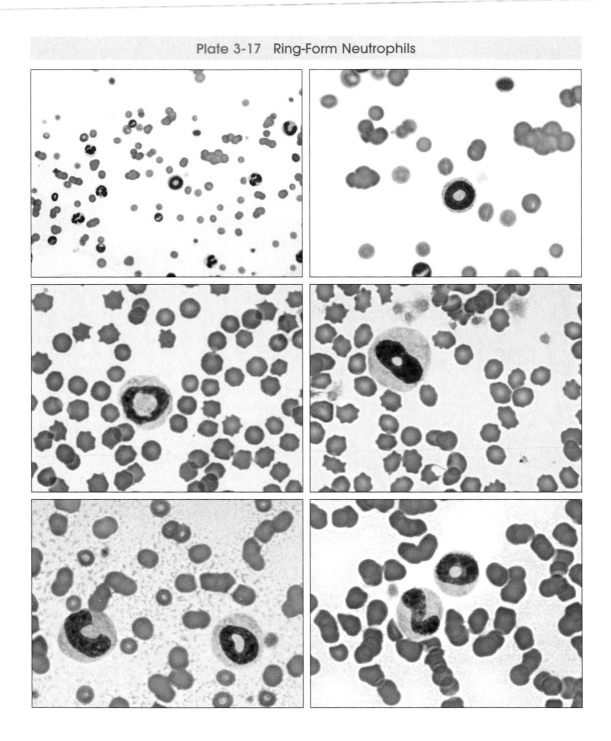

Plate 3-17   Ring-Form Neutrophils *(con't)*

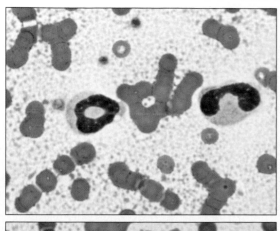
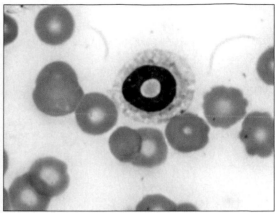
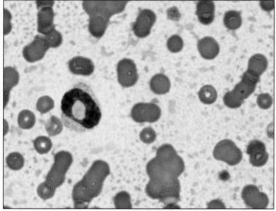

Giant Neutrophils

DISTINCTIVE FEATURES: Giant (larger than normal) neutrophils and bands are considered a toxic change that affects cell size.

DIAGNOSTIC SIGNIFICANCE: Skipped cell divisions during accelerated neutrophil production and maturation process may lead to the formation of large neutrophils and bands in the peripheral blood. This is generally associated with other toxic changes.

> ***NEXT STEPS:*** Giant neutrophils and bands are usually associated with other toxic changes. If other evidence of toxicity is not present, then other causes of giant neutrophils, for example, poodle macrocytosis (poodle marrow dyscrasia syndrome), FeLV myelodysplasia in cats, and administration of certain chemotherapeutics, should be investigated.

Plate 3-18   Giant Neutrophils

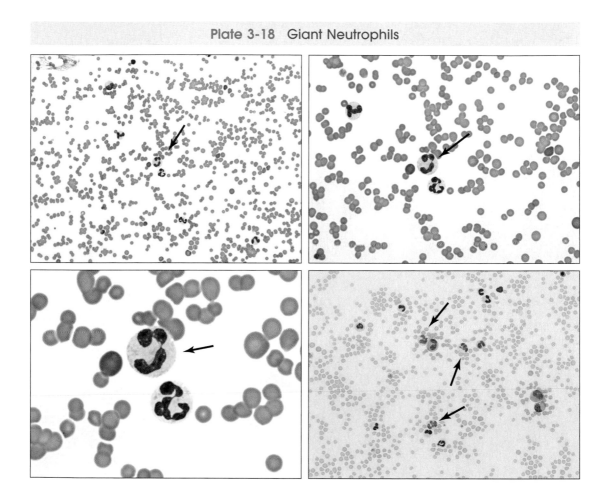

Plate 3-18 Giant Neutrophils *(con't)*

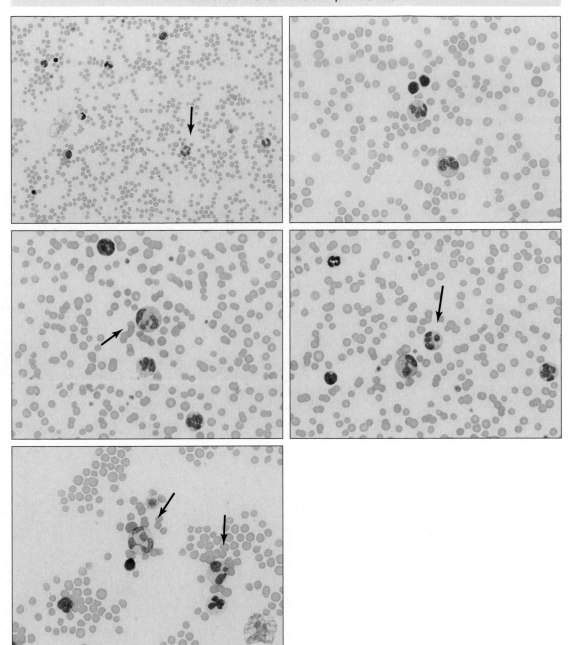

Lymphocytes

Lymphocytes vary in size in the peripheral blood of dogs and cats. Small lymphocytes predominate with a few lymphocytes that are slightly to moderately larger. Larger lymphocytes in peripheral blood have less densely staining, but still clearly clumped, nuclear chromatin. Lymphocytes are typically the second most common peripheral blood leukocyte (mature neutrophil being the most common).

Small Lymphocytes

DISTINCTIVE FEATURES: Small lymphocytes are mature cells, approximately 10 µm in diameter with densely staining (dark purple), round to oval nuclei, which are sometimes slightly indented and usually have large, well-defined chromatin clumps (heterochromatin) with intermixed smooth glassy areas (euchromatin). Occasionally, small lymphocytes may have nuclear chromatin, which appears smudged, especially with quick stains. The nucleus is eccentric, and a scant amount of moderately blue cytoplasm exists. Because of the eccentric placement of the nucleus, it is difficult to completely trace the rim of cytoplasm around the nucleus.

DIAGNOSTIC SIGNIFICANCE: Small lymphocytes are the most abundant form of lymphocyte in canine and feline blood. Increased numbers (lymphocytosis) may occur with epinephrine release secondary to excitement (mild lymphocytosis is common in young dogs and cats); chronic immune stimulation, and lymphoid neoplasia (chronic lymphocytic leukemia). Decreased numbers (lymphopenia) of lymphocytes may occur with acute inflammation or, commonly, as a "stress" leukogram secondary to glucocorticoid release.

> **NEXT STEPS:** Be careful to not confuse small lymphocytes with nucleated red blood cells such as rubricytes and metarubricytes. A rim of cytoplasm may usually be traced entirely around the nucleus of nucleated RBCs but not in mature lymphocytes.

Distinguishing a lymphocytosis secondary to immunostimulation from chronic lymphocytic leukemia may be difficult. Careful assessment for underlying infectious disease (especially ehrlichiosis in dogs), correlation of the age of the patient and clinical signs (chronic lymphocytic leukemia is uncommon in young animals), serial monitoring of lymphocyte absolute numbers and morphology, and, in some cases, the use of adjunct diagnostics (immunostains and flow cytometry) should be employed.

Plate 3-19 Small Mature Lymphocytes

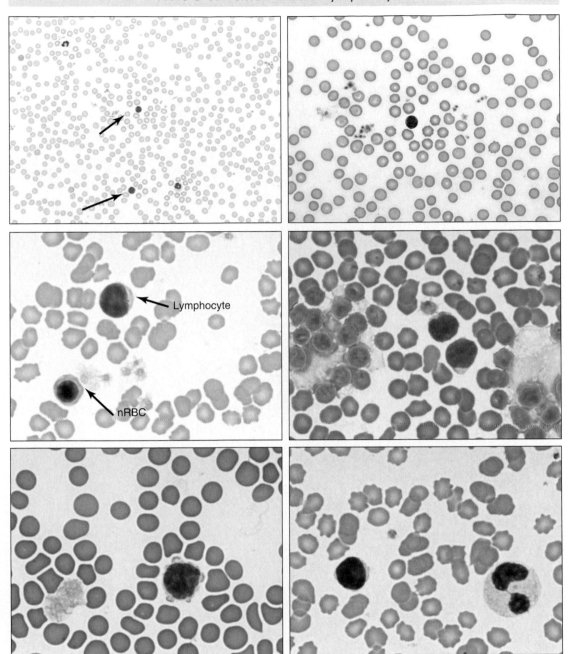

Plate 3-19 Small Mature Lymphocytes *(con't)*

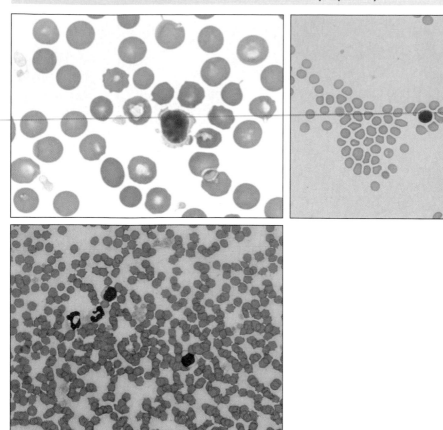

A, Small mature lymphocyte. Note eccentric nucleus and scant rim of cytoplasm **B,** Nucleated red blood cell. Note cytoplasm surrounding the more central nucleus

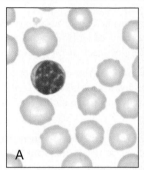
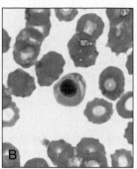

Reactive Lymphocytes

DISTINCTIVE FEATURES: The primary features that identify a reactive lymphocyte are cytoplasmic changes. In general, reactive lymphocytes are larger because of a mild to moderate increase in the amount of cytoplasm, and the cytoplasm stains more deeply basophilic compared with the cytoplasm of small, mature lymphocytes. Additionally, the nuclear chromatin is less condensed. The deep cytoplasmic basophilia of reactive lymphocytes represents an abundance of polyribosomes associated with increased protein synthesis and usually contrasts with the pale, perinuclear Golgi region.

DIAGNOSTIC SIGNIFICANCE: Reactive lymphocytes are immune-stimulated lymphocytes with upregulated synthesis of inflammatory mediators, and/or immunoglobulins (antibodies), or both. Reactive lymphocytes in peripheral blood suggest active, systemic antigenic stimulation secondary to both infectious and noninfectious disorders.

NEXT STEPS: It is important to differentiate reactive lymphocytes from neoplastic lymphocytes. In general, reactive lymphocytes occurring secondary to systemic immune stimulation, are present together with a wide range of lymphocyte morphology (small, mature lymphocytes; reactive lymphocytes; plasmacytoid lymphocytes; intermediate-sized lymphocytes; and occasionally also granular lymphocytes). Neoplastic lymphocytes, as discussed in Section V: Hematopoietic Neoplasia, may be small, intermediate sized, and blastic. If in high numbers, neoplastic lymphocytes are morphologically similar, forming a uniform population. Further testing such as immunostaining and flow cytometry may be needed to identify a neoplastic population of lymphocytes.

Plate 3-20   Reactive Lymphocytes

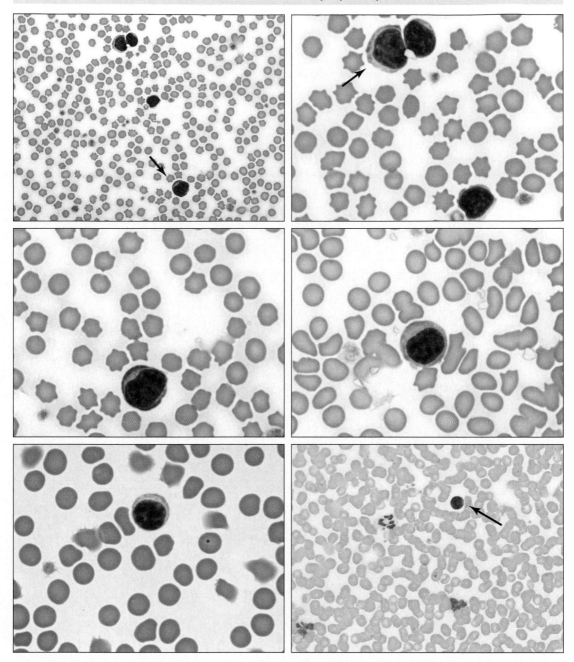

Plasmacytoid Reactive Lymphocytes

DISTINCTIVE FEATURES: With strong, chronic inflammation, reactive lymphocytes may become plasmacytoid (plasma cells in peripheral blood). Plasma cells are well differentiated B lymphocytes. They are larger than small lymphocytes and have an eccentrically placed round nucleus, with condensed nuclear chromatin and deeply basophilic cytoplasm because of the abundant polyribosomes associated with increased protein synthesis. Also, a perinuclear clear zone (Golgi region) is generally visible.

DIAGNOSTIC SIGNIFICANCE: Plasmacytoid reactive lymphocytes indicate strong, chronic, systemic inflammation but are etiologically nonspecific.

> **NEXT STEPS:** If significant numbers of plasmacytoid lymphocytes are present, investigate for infectious or inflammatory disease, rule out recent vaccination, and, if associated with hyperglobulinemia, consider serum electrophoresis to characterize the immunoglobulin pattern, which aids in categorizing the inflammatory response and may also be used to check for lymphoid malignancy (lymphoid leukemia, plasma cell neoplasia, lymphoma).

Plate 3-21 Plasmacytoid Reactive Lymphocytes

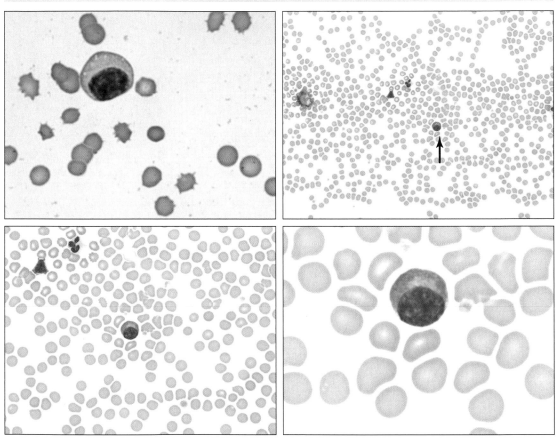

Plate 3-21   Plasmacytoid Reactive Lymphocytes *(con't)*

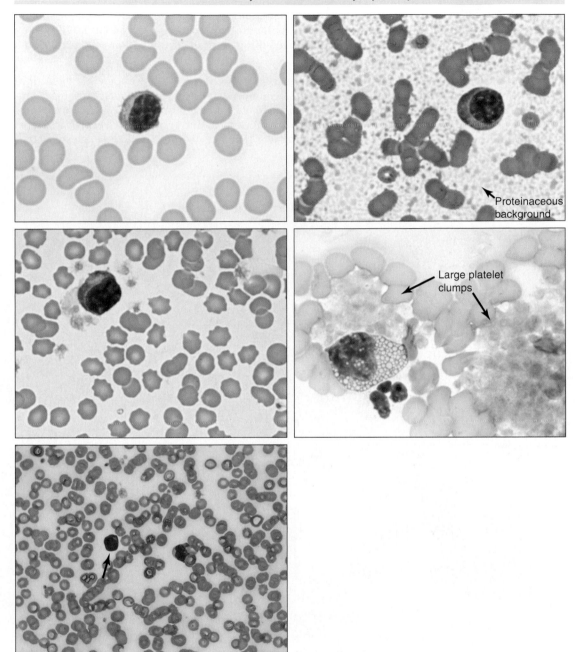

Proteinaceous background

Large platelet clumps

Granular Lymphocytes (Large Granular Lymphocytes)

DISTINCTIVE FEATURES: Large granular lymphocytes have a slightly larger nucleus and moderate amount of cytoplasm, which ranges from light to moderately basophilic and contains few, variably sized, eosinophilic intracytoplasmic granules that may be dispersed throughout the cytoplasm or concentrated in a perinuclear region of the cytoplasm.

DIAGNOSTIC SIGNIFICANCE: Large granular lymphocytes may be present in low numbers in the peripheral blood of clinically normal dogs and cats. Increased numbers may occur with chronic immune stimulation (especially chronic ehrlichiosis in dogs). When moderate to high numbers of granular lymphocytes are present in peripheral blood and infectious disease has been ruled out, granular lymphocytic leukemia or circulating neoplastic cells from lymphoma of granular lymphocyte origin should be investigated.

Plate 3-22   Granular Lymphocytes

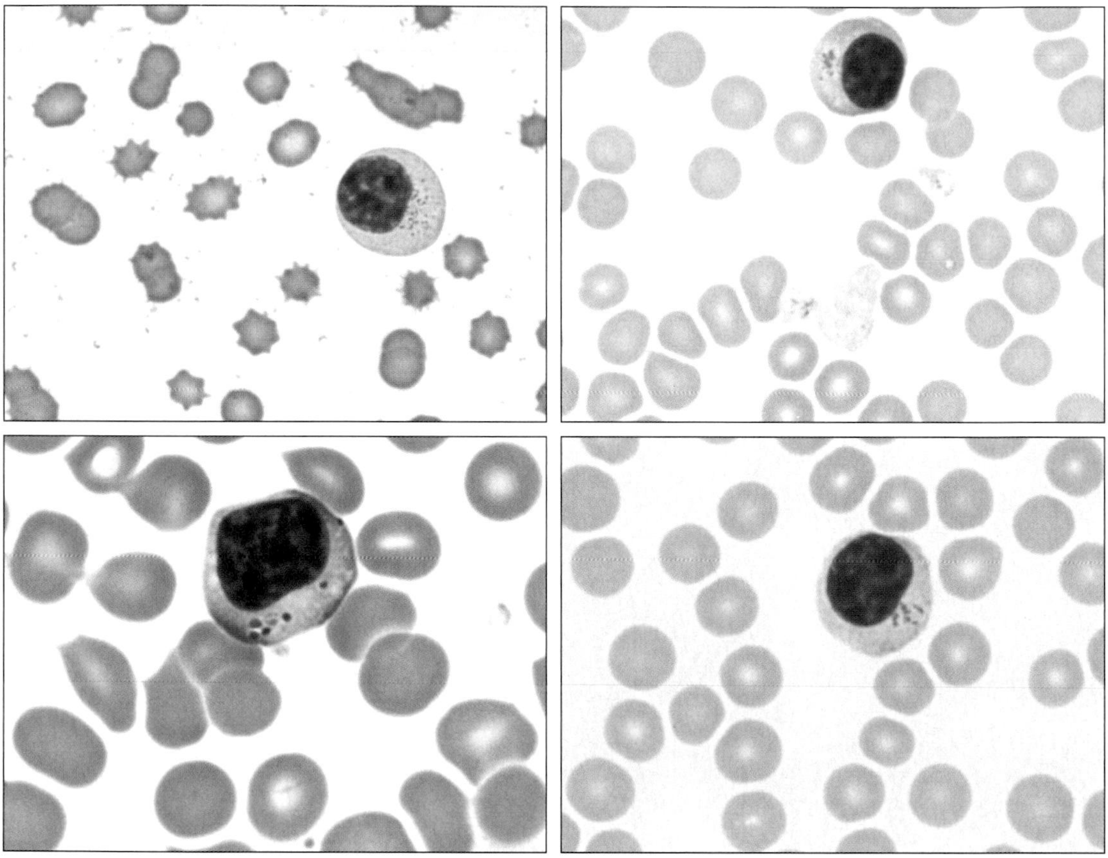

Plate 3-22 Granular Lymphocytes *(con't)*

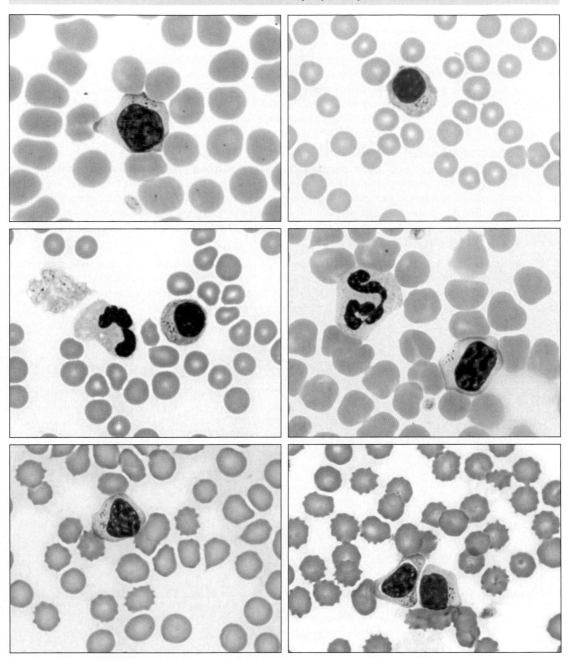

Monocytes

DISTINCTIVE FEATURES: Canine and feline monocytes are larger than neutrophils and similar in size or slightly larger than eosinophils and basophils. Their nuclei vary greatly in morphology, ranging from elongated U-shapes that resemble band neutrophils to irregular multilobulated forms. The nuclear chromatin is characteristically lacy to ropy, with only a few small isolated clumps of heterochromatin. The cytoplasm is moderate to abundant, gray-blue with a ground-glass texture, often sparsely dusted with minute eosinophilic granules, and occasionally lightly vacuolated. Cytoplasmic borders are usually irregular, sometimes with fine, filamentous, pseudopodia-like extensions. Because of their relatively large size, monocytes may be concentrated along the feathered edge, and their proportion underestimated in blood smear differential white blood cell (WBC) counts.

DIAGNOSTIC SIGNIFICANCE: A few monocytes are present in the peripheral blood of healthy dogs and cats. Increased numbers of monocytes (monocytosis) may occur with disorders such as subacute and chronic inflammation, excess endogenous or exogenous glucocorticoids (common in the dog but inconsistent in the cat), autoimmune hemolytic anemia (part of a leukemoid response to accelerated hematopoiesis), FIV infection (cat), and neoplasia of the monocytic cell line (rare). Decreased numbers of monocytes (monocytopenia) is not diagnostically significant because of the normally low numbers of monocytes in healthy dogs and cats.

In conditions such as severe bacterial infections or septicemia, some of the circulating monocytes may have transformed into macrophages. Macrophages are often highly vacuolated with an increased amount of lightly basophilic cytoplasm and convoluted nuclei. Sometimes, these cells are referred to as *reactive* or *toxic monocytes* and yet are very rarely identified in peripheral blood.

Plate 3-23   Monocytes

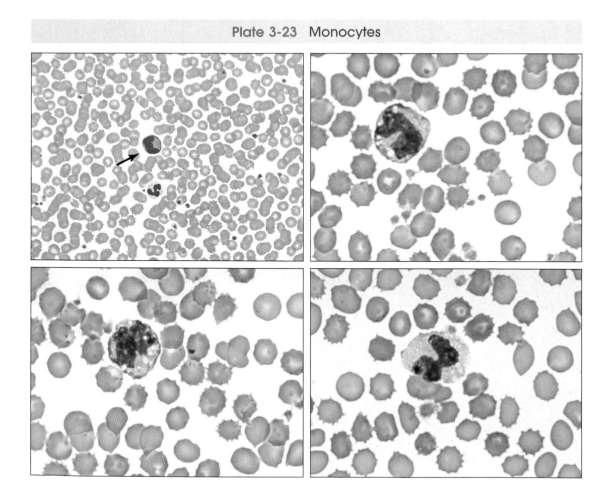

Plate 3-23 Monocytes *(con't)*

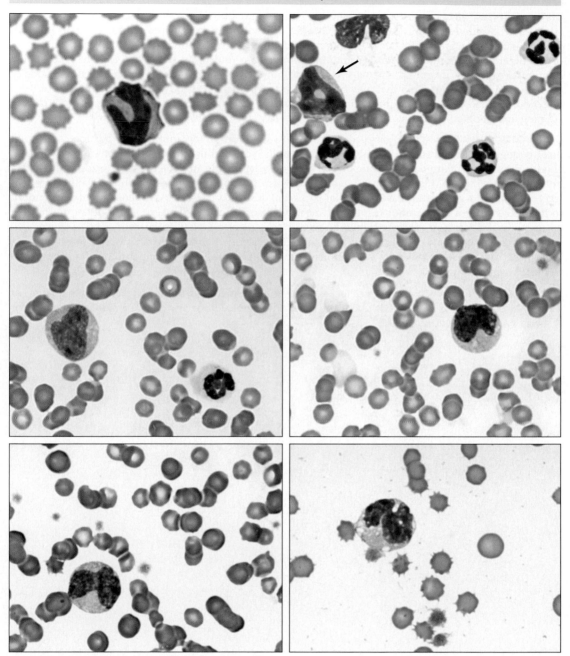

Eosinophils

DISTINCTIVE FEATURES: Eosinophils are slightly larger than neutrophils, with nuclei that are less lobulated, often divided into only two distinct lobules, and with less condensed chromatin than those of mature neutrophils. The cytoplasm of eosinophils is clear to faintly basophilic and contains large numbers of prominent pink granules. Feline eosinophil granules are uniformly small and rod shaped. Canine eosinophil granules are round and vary widely in number and size. Canine eosinophils occasionally contain a single, large granule that may be mistaken for an inclusion body or organism. Eosinophils of Greyhounds (and few other Sight Hound breeds) are peculiar because they may degranulate during staining and appear vacuolated on smears (the so-called *gray eosinophils of Greyhounds*).

DIAGNOSTIC SIGNIFICANCE: Eosinophils may usually be found in low numbers in the blood smears of healthy dogs and cats. Increased numbers of eosinophils (eosinophilia) may occur with many hypersensitivity diseases of allergic or parasitic origin, both of which could involve the skin (ectoparasites, flea bite dermatitis), lungs (heartworm infection, lungworm infection, feline asthma), and gastrointestinal tract (inflammatory bowel disease, intestinal parasites). Rarely, a paraneoplastic eosinophilia secondary to the presence of a solid tumor (especially mast cell neoplasia) may be seen. A moderate to marked eosinophilia, which is unexplained, may be seen with eosinophilic leukemia (rare). Excess glucocorticoids, either endogenous or exogenous, may cause a decrease in circulating eosinophils (eosinopenia). Otherwise, due to low numbers of eosinophils normally in the dog and cat, an eosinopenia is not diagnostically significant.

NEXT STEPS: If an eosinophilia is detected, further assessment for underlying allergic, parasitic, or neoplastic disease is warranted. Check the blood film carefully for any circulating mast cells and for hemoparasites (microfilaria).

Plate 3-24   Canine Eosinophils

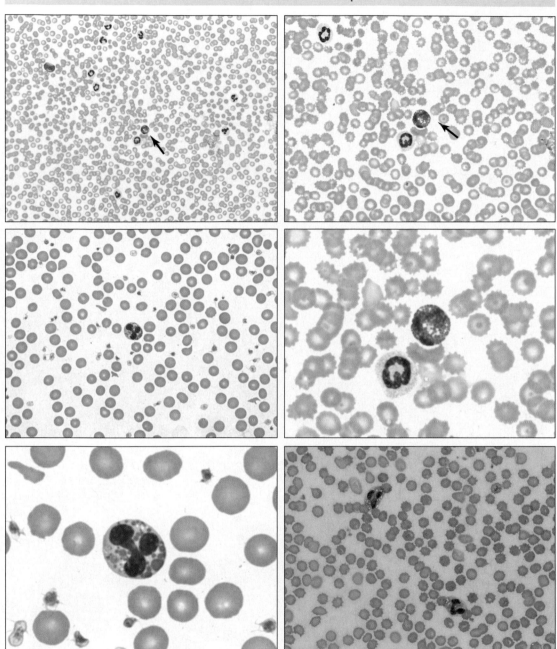

Plate 3-25   Feline Eosinophils

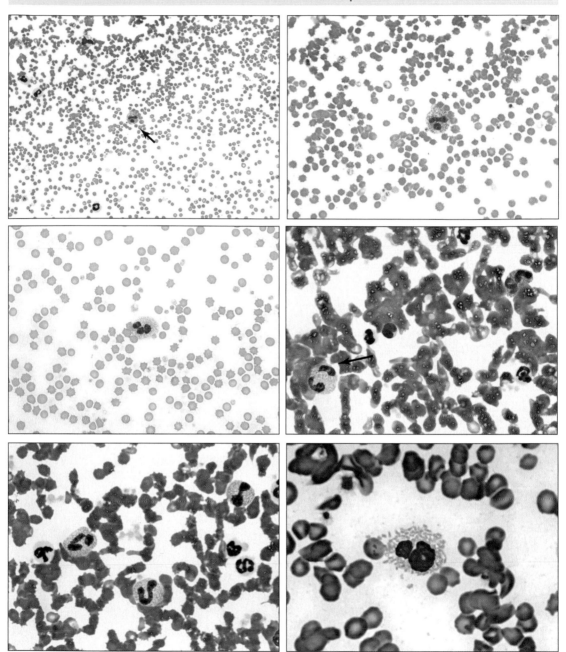

Plate 3-25 Feline Eosinophils *(con't)*

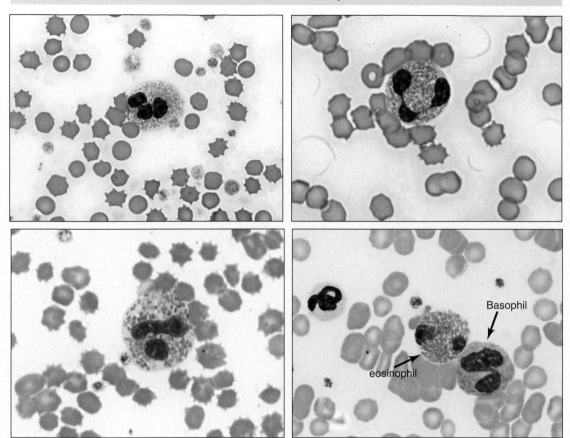

Plate 3-26 Grey Eosinophils of Sight Hounds

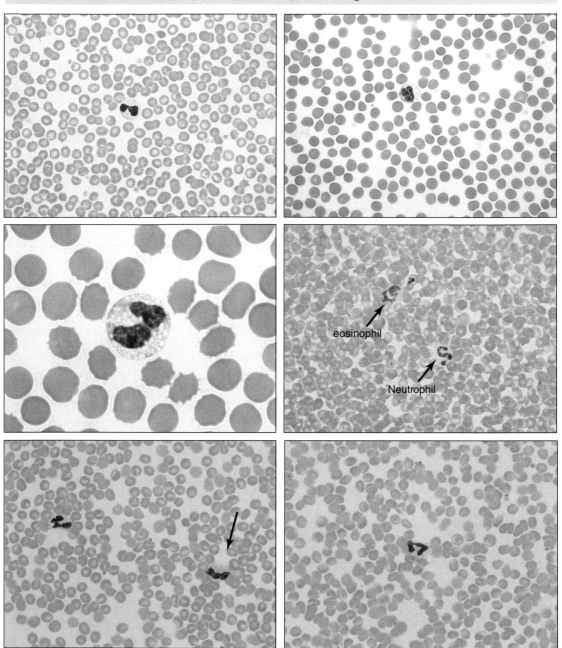

Plate 3-26 Grey Eosinophils of Sight Hounds *(con't)*

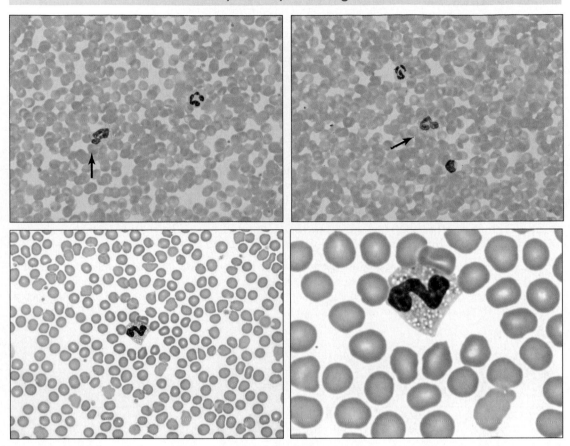

Basophils

DISTINCTIVE FEATURES: Basophils are the largest and least numerous of the mature granulocytic cell types and are often not seen on a standard 100-cell differential cell count in healthy dogs and cats. Basophil nuclei are less densely staining, have fewer lobulations, and have a more elongated, ribbonlike appearance compared with the nuclei of neutrophils. The basophil cytoplasm is pale to moderately blue-gray to purple and typically contains granules. Occasionally, no granules may be visible. Granule size and color vary between dogs and cats. In dogs, basophil granules are usually low in number (typically <50 granules per cell) and stain dark blue to metachromatic. Canine basophils occasionally lack obvious granules but are recognizable by their size, nuclear morphology, and cytoplasmic staining. In cats, basophils contain abundant oval, pale lavender to gray granules, although immature basophils may also contain a few primary, dark purple granules.

DIAGNOSTIC SIGNIFICANCE: Basophils are rare in the peripheral blood of healthy dogs and cats. Increased numbers of basophils (basophilia) are often associated with a concurrent eosinophilia, and similar etiologies of hypersensitivity disease as for increased eosinophils apply for a basophilia. A moderate to marked unexplained basophilia may occur secondary to basophilic leukemia (extremely rare). Decreased numbers of basophils (basopenia) are not diagnostically significant because of the low numbers of basophils in the peripheral blood of healthy dogs and cats.

> **NEXT STEPS:** Be careful to not confuse mast cells with basophils. Mast cells are larger than basophils and often will be found concentrated on the feathered edge of the smear. Mast cells usually contain large numbers of granules compared with basophils, and mast cell nuclei are round to ovoid, whereas basophil nuclei are ribbonlike.

Plate 3-27 Canine Basophils

Plate 3-27   Canine Basophils *(con't)*

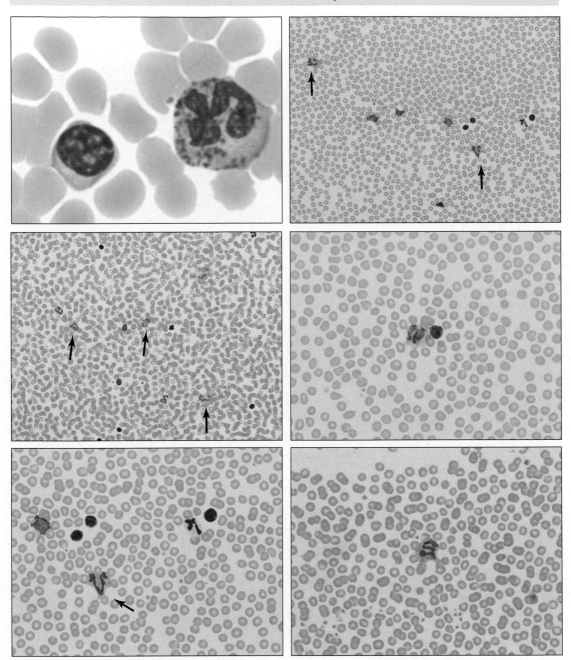

A, Canine basophil **B,** Canine mast cell

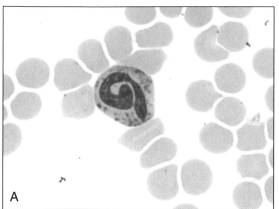
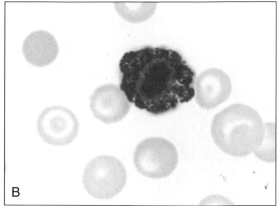

A

B

Plate 3-28 Feline Basophils

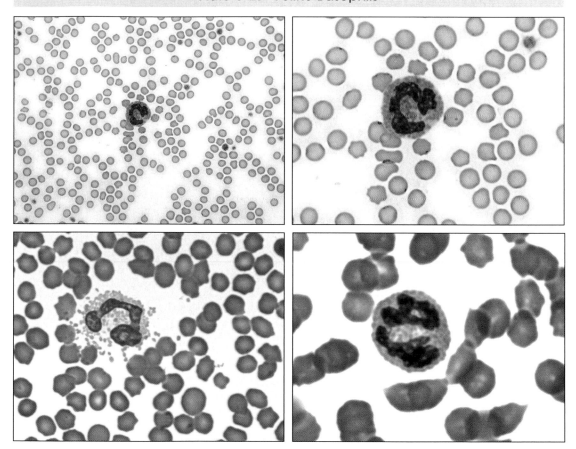

Plate 3-28 Feline Basophils *(con't)*

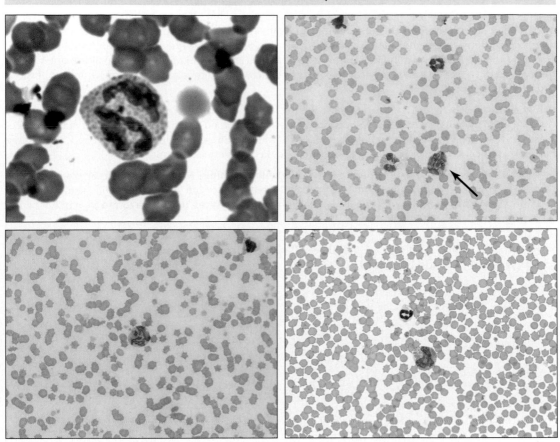

A, Feline basophil **B,** Feline mast cell

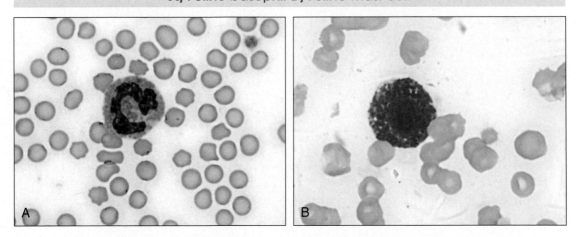

Mast Cells

DISTINCTIVE FEATURES: Mast cells are large mononuclear cells that have a moderate to abundant amount of pale blue cytoplasm. The nucleus is round to oval, and the cytoplasm contains many small, round, intensely staining, intracytoplasmic metachromatic (reddish-purple) granules. Granule numbers range from few to many, but typically high numbers of granules are present and may be so abundant as to fill the cytoplasm, obscuring the nucleus. Poorly differentiated mast cells may have low numbers of intracytoplasmic granules.

DIAGNOSTIC SIGNIFICANCE: Rarely, a mast cell may be seen on the peripheral blood smear of a healthy dog or cat. Mast cells have been observed in the peripheral blood of dogs and cats with mast cell neoplasia and in very low numbers on blood smears from dogs with severe inflammatory conditions. Large numbers of mast cells may be seen with mast cell leukemia (very uncommon).

NEXT STEPS: Be careful to not confuse mast cells with basophils. Mast cells are larger than basophils and often will be found concentrated on the feathered edge of the smear. Mast cells usually contain large numbers of granules compared with basophils, and mast cell nuclei are round to ovoid, whereas basophil nuclei are ribbonlike.

Finding circulating mast cells on peripheral blood smears from dogs and especially cats warrants a thorough search for underlying mast cell neoplasia of the skin, liver, spleen, and gastrointestinal tract.

Plate 3-29 Mast Cells

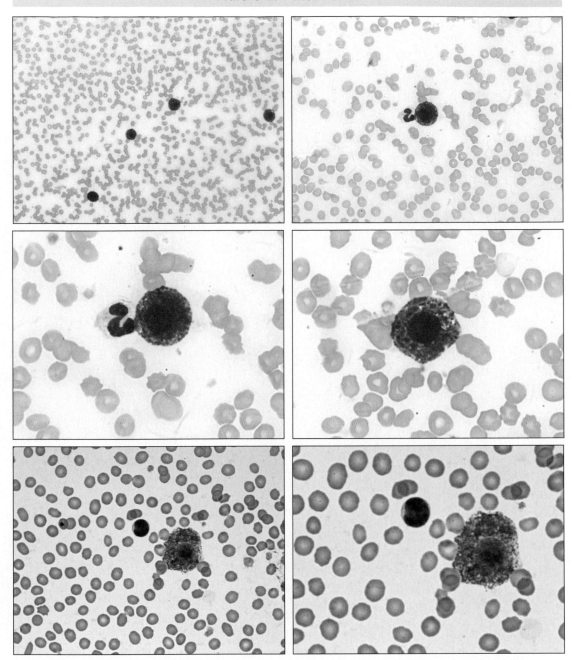

Plate 3-29 Mast Cells *(con't)*

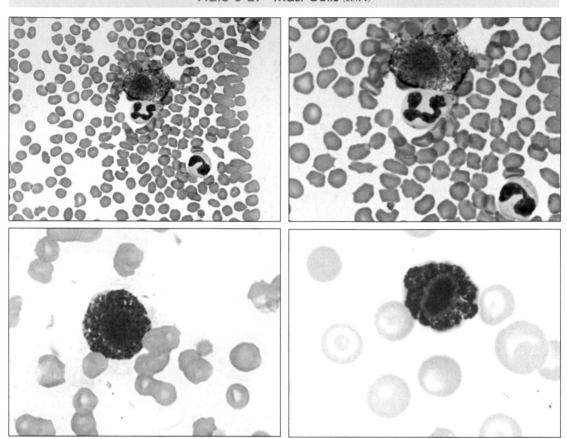

A, Feline basophil **B,** Feline mast cell

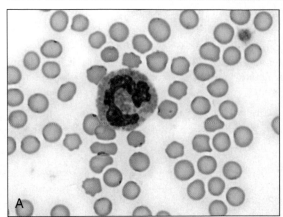

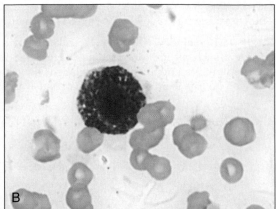

C, Canine basophil **D,** Canine mast cell

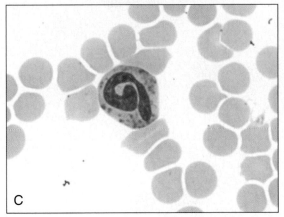

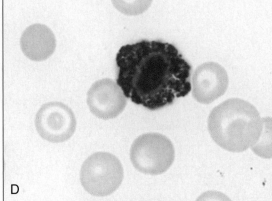

Sideroleukocytes

DISTINCTIVE FEATURES: Sideroleukocytes are neutrophils or monocytes containing intracytoplasmic, yellowish-brown to blue-black hemosiderin pigment.

DIAGNOSTIC SIGNIFICANCE: Sideroleukocytes are rarely observed on peripheral blood smears with disorders such as immune-mediated hemolytic anemia (IMHA) and following blood transfusions. Hemosiderin is an iron-containing pigment, and sideroleukocytes may be confirmed by staining a blood film with an iron stain such as Prussian blue (rarely done).

NEXT STEPS: If sideroleukocytes are identified and a blood transfusion has not been performed, top consideration is IMHA and warrants close review of the blood film for ghost RBCs, spherocytes, RBC agglutination, and hemoparasites.

Plate 3-30 Sideroleukocytes

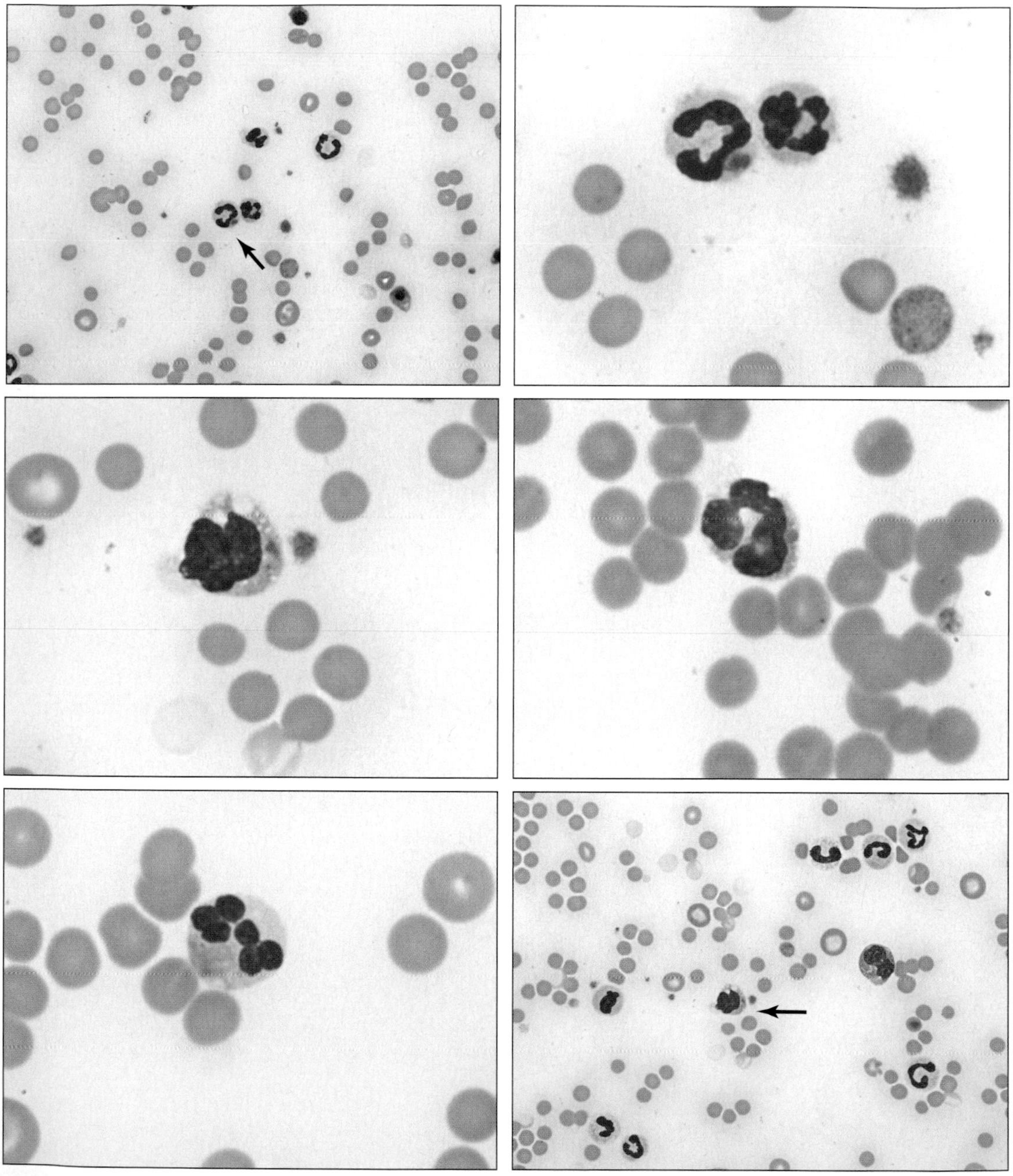

Plate 3-30   Sideroleukocytes *(con't)*

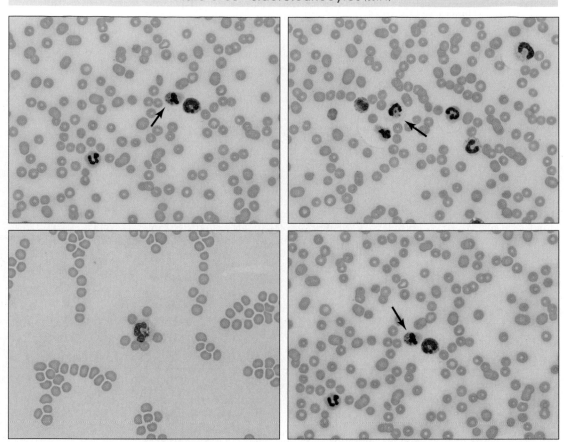

Erythrophage (Erythrophagocytosis)

DISTINCTIVE FEATURES: An erythrophage is a leukocyte (usually a neutrophil or monocyte) containing engulfed RBCs (erythrophagocytosis).

DIAGNOSTIC SIGNIFICANCE: Erythrophagocytosis is uncommonly identified on peripheral blood smears and may be observed with immune-mediated diseases and some leukemias.

Plate 3-31 Erythrophages

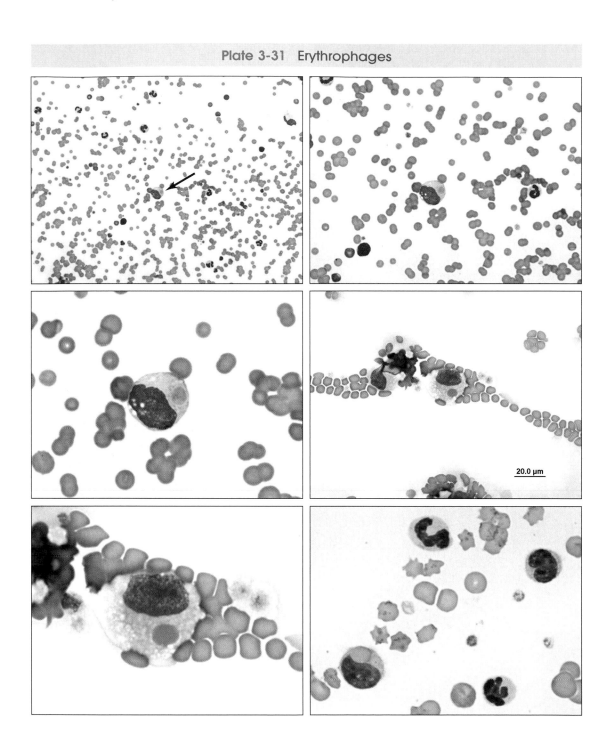

Plate 3-31 Erythrophages *(con't)*

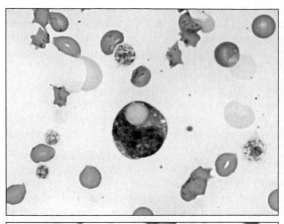

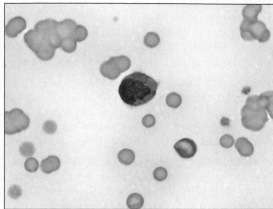

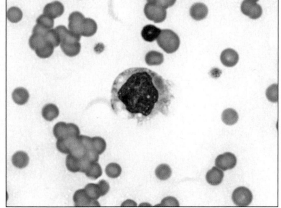

Macrophage

DISTINCTIVE FEATURES: Macrophages are inflammatory cells found in tissue and only very uncommonly in the peripheral blood of healthy dogs and cats. Macrophages are large mononuclear cells with abundant clear cytoplasm and round nuclei with coarse chromatin and are often vacuolated and sometimes cytophagic. They may be uniform but, in some neoplastic conditions, may have criteria of malignancy (large cell and nuclear size, multiple nuclei, prominent nucleoli).

DIAGNOSTIC SIGNIFICANCE: Monocytes are the peripheral blood precursors to tissue macrophages. Monocytes leave peripheral blood secondary to inflammatory mediators and develop into tissue macrophages. Macrophages have phagocytic activity and may engulf foreign material, cells, infectious agents (especially fungal organisms), and debris. If macrophages are found in peripheral blood smears, they are usually on the feathered edge because of their large size.

> **NEXT STEPS:** Macrophages are rarely found in the peripheral blood of healthy animals; however, when collecting blood from a patient, if a regional source of inflammation or infection is present, concurrent sampling of subcutaneous tissue may occasionally result in low numbers of tissue macrophages in blood. If macrophages demonstrate criteria of malignancy, then histiocytic neoplasia should be strongly suspected and would warrant assessment for histiocytic neoplasia of the lymph nodes, liver, spleen, lungs, and bone marrow.

Plate 3-32 Macrophages

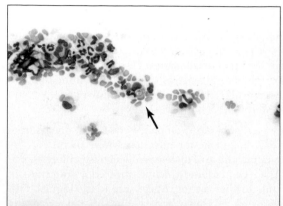

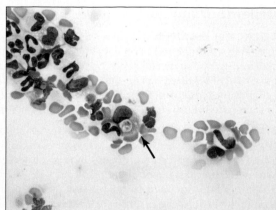

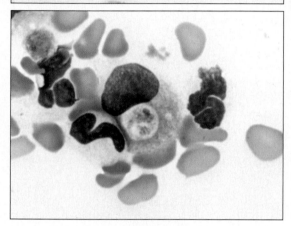

Inclusions, Parasites, and Infectious Agents

Distemper Inclusions

DISTINCTIVE FEATURES: Distemper inclusions are aggregates of viral nucleocapsids that appear as round to oval to irregular, red to blue, cytoplasmic structures. The inclusions tend to occur in either the monocyte and lymphocyte cell series or the neutrophil and erythrocyte cell series. Distemper inclusions are most easily identified on Diff-Quik–stained smears as bright, homogeneous, eosinophilic, round to ovoid cytoplasmic structures. Distemper inclusions may be seen on Wright-stained smears; however, they tend to stain pale blue and are somewhat more difficult to identify.

DIAGNOSTIC SIGNIFICANCE: Distemper inclusions are seen only rarely on peripheral blood smears from dogs with distemper; however, when present, they are diagnostic for infection. These inclusions are found in a small percentage of dogs during the acute viremic phase of distemper, which is usually associated with clinical signs of upper respiratory disease. The lack of identifiable inclusions does not rule out distemper infection, and if suspected clinically, warrants further testing. Make sure to distinguish Distemper inclusions from other inclusions and artifacts such as Döhle bodies, Ehrlichia morulae and platelets overlying WBCs.

Plate 3-33   Distemper Inclusions

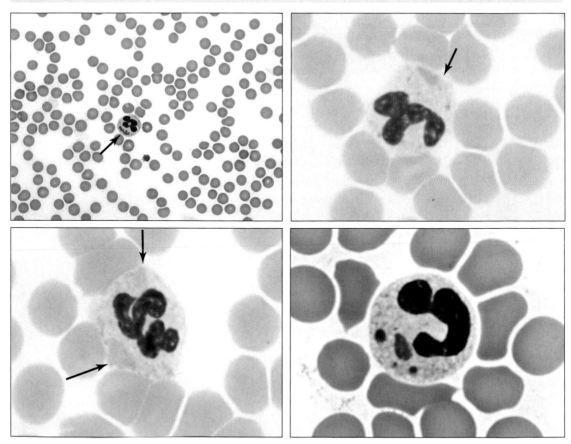

Plate 3-33 Distemper Inclusions *(con't)*

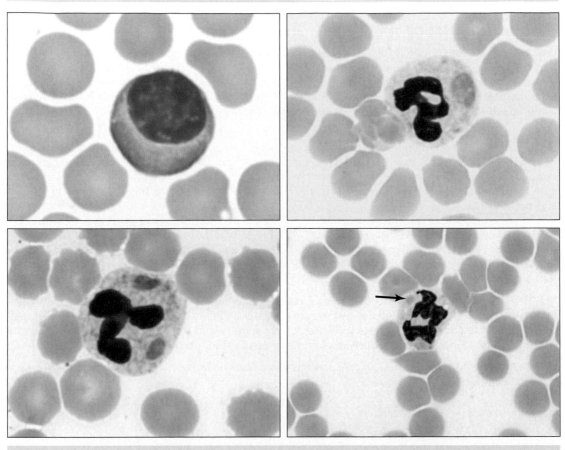

A, Döhle bodies **B,** Canine neutrophil with *Ehrlichia* morulae
C, Distemper inclusions **D,** Platelet over neutrophil

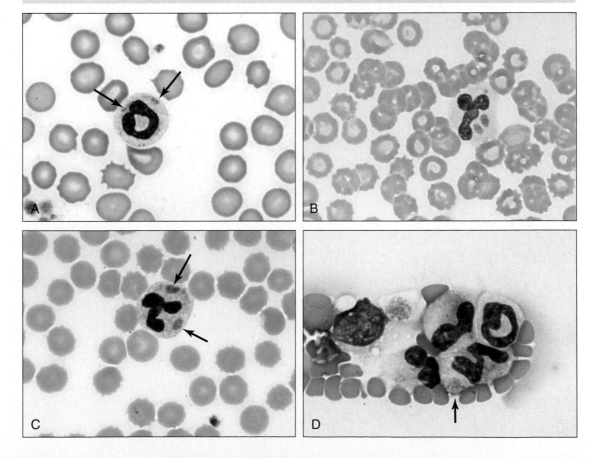

Ehrlichia/Anaplasma **spp.**

DISTINCTIVE FEATURES: Ehrlichiosis is a group of tickborne diseases caused by a gram-negative intracellular bacterium that infects blood cells. The disease is categorized by the host and the type of blood cell infected. On light microscopy, *Ehrlichia* organisms form aggregates within a cytoplasmic vacuole called a *morula*. Morulae are large, round to oval clusters composed of small dotlike organisms, which stain as a stippled dark blue inclusion. One or more morulae may be present in a cell.

Canine monocytic ehrlichiosis is caused primarily by *Ehrlichia canis* and less commonly by *Ehrlichia chaffeensis*. Morulae are found primarily within the cytoplasm of monocytes. The disease may be acute or chronic. Clinical signs may be mild to severe and may include fever, lethargy, anorexia, enlarged lymph nodes and spleen, bleeding disorders, vomiting or diarrhea, ocular changes, and neurologic signs. CBC abnormalities may include one or all of the following: nonregenerative anemia, thrombocytopenia, and neutropenia.

Canine granulocytic ehrlichiosis is caused by *Ehrlichia ewingii* and *Anaplasma phagocytophilum* (formerly *Ehrlichia equi* and *Ehrlichia phagocytophilia*). Morulae are found primarily in the cytoplasm of neutrophils. Disease, clinical signs, and CBC changes are essentially the same as in canine monocytic ehrlichiosis; however, suppurative polyarthritis is more commonly seen with granulocytic ehrlichiosis. Rare cases of cats infected with *Anaplasma phagocytophilum* have been documented.

DIAGNOSTIC SIGNIFICANCE: Identification of morulae is diagnostic for ehrlichiosis or anaplasmosis. However, morulae are not seen in the vast majority of cases and may be present in low numbers of cells. If infection is suspected, further testing (serology, polymerase chain reaction [PCR]) may be needed for diagnosis. Also, further testing for other tickborne disease is recommended to rule out co-infections.

NEXT STEPS: Be careful to not confuse artifacts (i.e., platelet overlying leukocyte) or other inclusions (i.e., Döhle bodies) with morulae.

Plate 3-34 *Ehrlichia* Morula

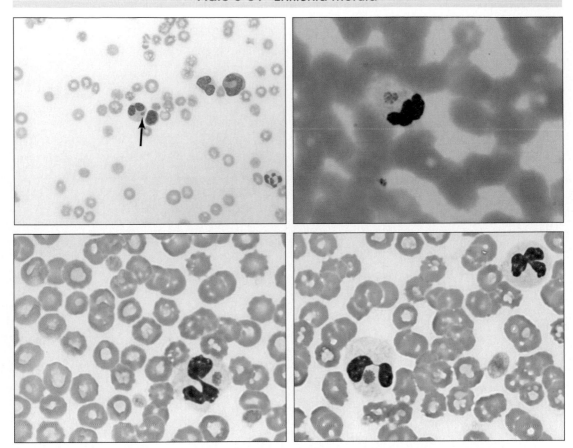

Plate 3-34   *Ehrlichia* Morula *(con't)*

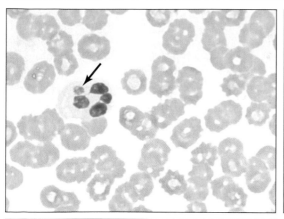
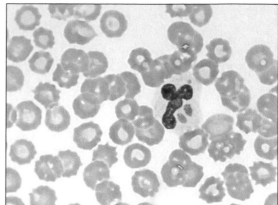

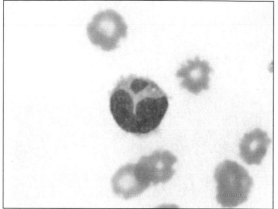

A, Döhle bodies **B,** Canine neutrophil with *Ehrlichia* morulae
C, Distemper inclusions **D,** Platelet over neutrophil

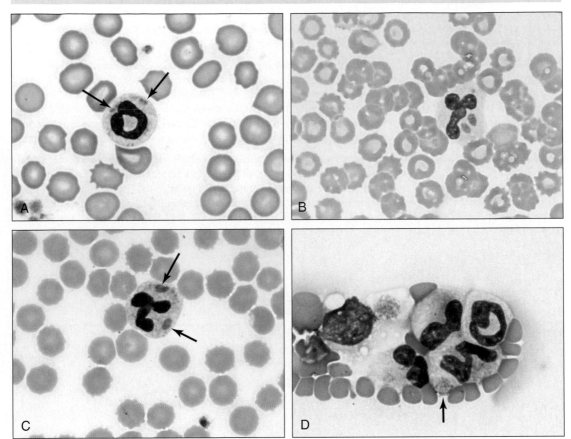

Hepatozoon spp.

DISTINCTIVE FEATURES: *Hepatozoon* spp. are protozoan parasites of dogs, with infection resulting from ingestion of infected ticks. The organism forms large (up to 11 µm) gametocytes, which are oval to elliptical, clear to pale blue structures within the cytoplasm of neutrophils, monocytes, or both. The organism typically displaces the nucleus to one side of the cell.

DIAGNOSTIC SIGNIFICANCE: Hepatozoonosis is caused by *Hepatozoon canis* and *Hepatozoon americanum* and is a severe disease that often results in death. Clinical signs are related to severe cardiac and skeletal muscle infection (myositis), with clinical signs that include fever, weight loss, muscle loss or wasting, and skeletal pain. CBC findings are often remarkable, as hepatozoonosis is frequently associated with a marked mature neutrophilic leukocytosis with or without a left shift. Gametocytes of *H. canis* are seldom found in peripheral blood leukocytes; however, gametocytes of *H. americanum* are frequently present.

NEXT STEPS: Identification of gametocytes in the cytoplasm of canine peripheral blood neutrophils and monocytes is diagnostic for hepatozoonosis. Lack of identification of the parasite does not rule out infection. If appropriate history of tick exposure, geographic location of the patient (most often seen in the Gulf Coast states of North America), appropriate clinical signs, and marked neutrophilia are present, further testing such as PCR should be performed.

Plate 3-35   *Hepatozoon* Gametocytes

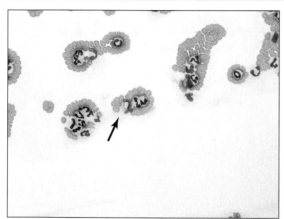
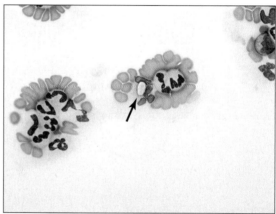
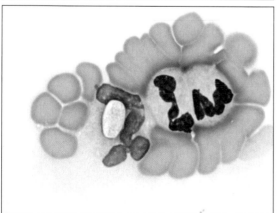
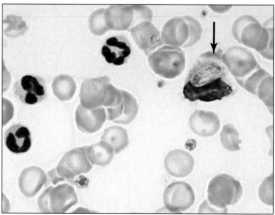

Plate 3-35   *Hepatozoon* Gametocytes *(con't)*

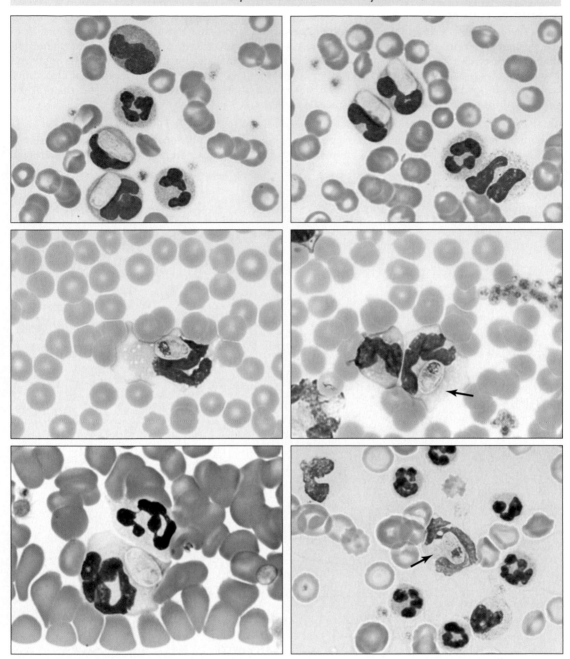

Histoplasma capsulatum

DISTINCTIVE FEATURES: *Histoplasma capsulatum* organisms are small (2 to 4 μm in diameter), round to oval yeast organisms found in the cytoplasm of peripheral blood monocytes, neutrophils, and occasionally eosinophils in infected dogs and cats. The yeasts have an eccentrically placed, reddish, crescent-shaped nucleus; clear to light blue cytoplasm; and a thin, clear halo (cell wall) surrounding the organism. The leukocytes typically show marked toxic changes. A cell may contain one or more yeast organisms, which may be seen extracellularly (free in the background of the smear) when leukocytes containing the yeast organisms have ruptured (during smear preparation).

DIAGNOSTIC SIGNIFICANCE: The presence of *Histoplasma* yeast organisms in peripheral blood indicates disseminated histoplasmosis and carries a poor prognosis. Localized histoplasmosis such as gastrointestinal histoplasmosis may become disseminated, especially if immunosuppressive doses of glucocorticoids are given.

Plate 3-36 *Histoplasma* Yeast

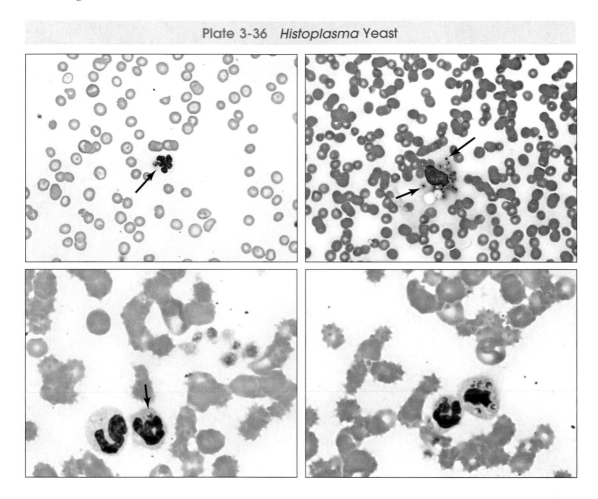

Plate 3-36   *Histoplasma* Yeast *(con't)*

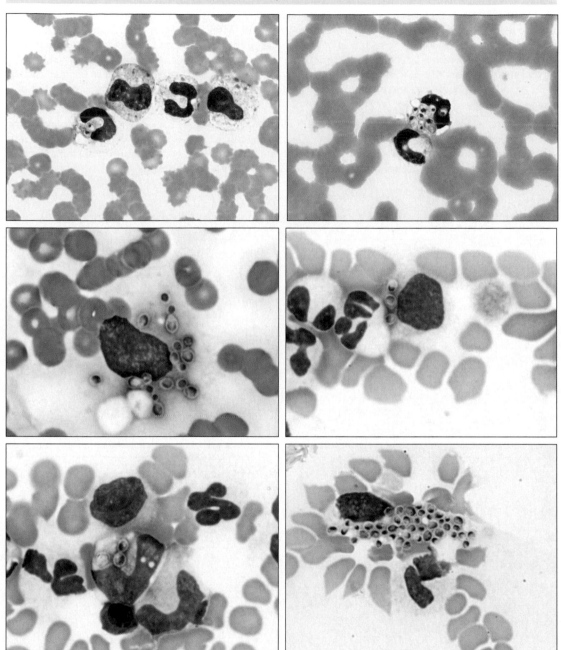

Mucopolysaccharidosis

DISTINCTIVE FEATURES: Mucopolysaccharidoses (MPSs) are a group of uncommon hereditary lysosomal storage disorders, which result in leukocyte inclusions. With MPS, the vast majority (generally ≥90%) of neutrophils, and occasionally also lymphocytes, contain reddish to purple intracytoplasmic granules. Basophils generally have larger granules, and in cats, basophil granules stain basophilic instead of the typical mauve color. Affected individuals often have significant physical abnormalities such as dished faces, small head and ears, and skeletal deformities of the spine and long bones, which are noted at a young age.

DIAGNOSTIC SIGNIFICANCE: MPS is generally associated with severe medical consequences in the homozygous state and a shortened life span. The cytoplasmic granules need to be distinguished from other granule abnormalities and from toxic granulation in neutrophils, normal neutrophil primary granules (usually very faint), Birman cat anomaly and Chédiak-Higashi syndrome.

Plate 3-37 Cytoplasmic Granules Associated with Mucopolysaccharidosis

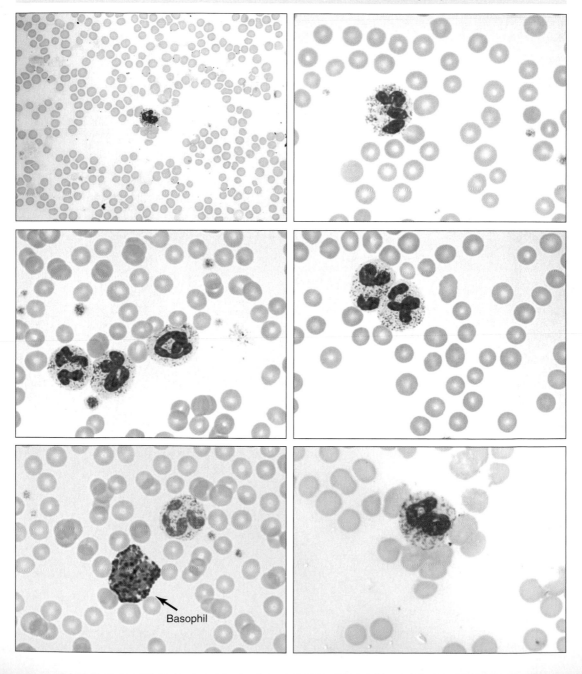

Basophil

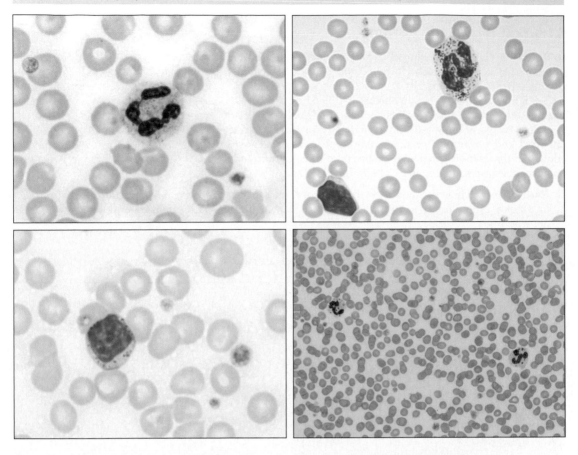

A, Toxic granulation **B,** Mucopolysaccharidosis **C,** Birman Cat Anomaly
D, Chédiak-Higashi Syndrome **E,** Primary neutrophil granules

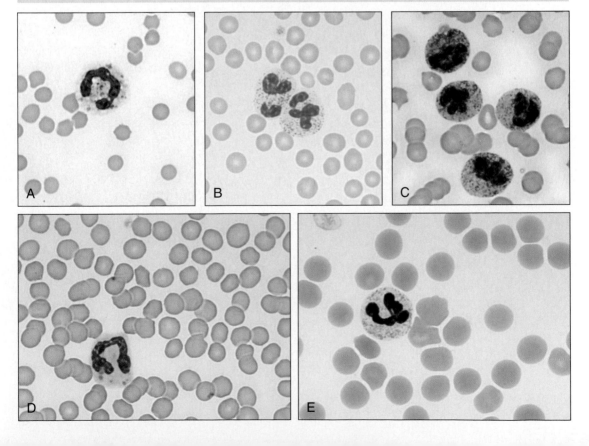

Chédiak-Higashi Syndrome

DISTINCTIVE FEATURES: Chédiak-Higashi syndrome (CHS) is a rare inherited disease found in smoke blue Persian cats, in which abnormal formation of lysosomal granules and abnormal degranulation occurs. Affected cats typically have a diluted smoke blue coat color and yellow-green irises and may have slight neutrophil function defects and bleeding disorders. With CHS, eosinophilic intracytoplasmic granules are found in neutrophils and less commonly in monocytes and lymphocytes. Leukocytes often contain a single granule but may contain two or three granules. Eosinophil and basophil granules are enlarged and eosinophil granules may appear roundish instead of having the typical rod shape. To confirm if the granules are Döhle bodies or granules associated with CHS, a blood smear may be stained using peroxidase staining, and CHS granules will stain black.

> **NEXT STEPS:** CHS is diagnosed on the basis of finding characteristic eosinophilic leukocyte granules in smoke blue Persian cats and ruling out other granule abnormalities and toxic change of neutrophils.

Plate 3-38 Cytoplasmic Granules Associated with Chédiak-Higashi Syndrome

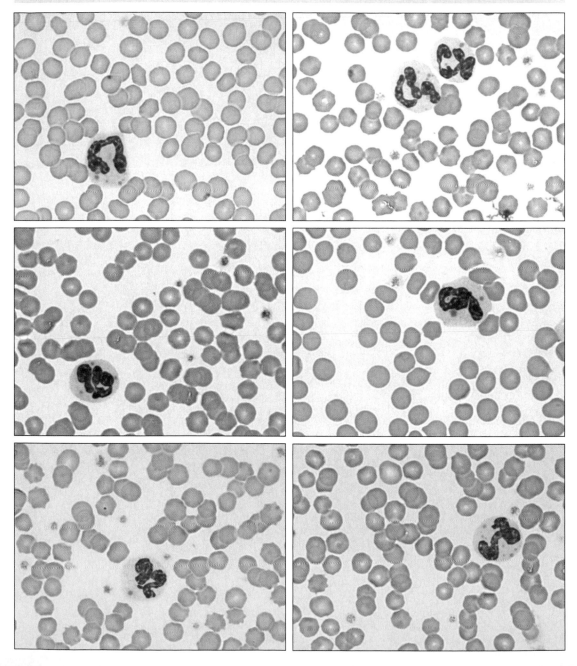

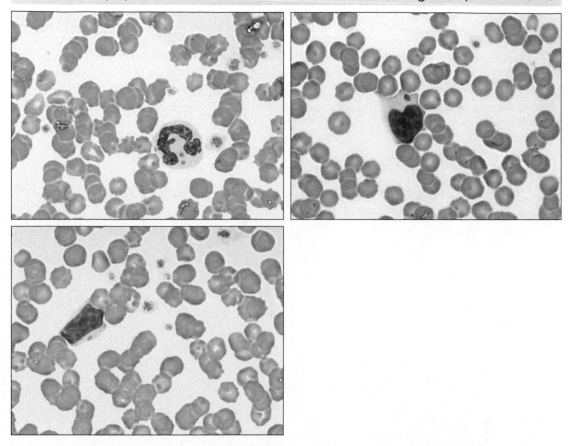

A, Toxic granulation **B,** Mucopolysaccharidosis **C,** Birman Cat Anomaly
D, Chédiak-Higashi Syndrome **E,** Primary neutrophil granules

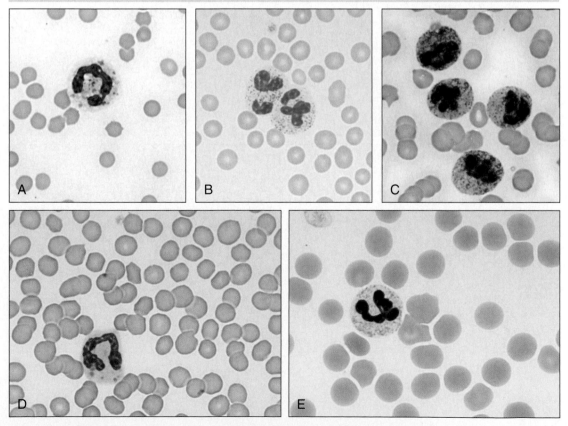

Birman Cat Anomaly

DISTINCTIVE FEATURES: Birman cat anomaly is an inherited neutrophil granulation defect of Birman cats with no clinical signs or evidence of neutrophil dysfunction. Fine eosinophilic granules are found in the cytoplasm of neutrophils.

DIAGNOSTIC SIGNIFICANCE: Birman cat anomaly must be differentiated from toxic granulation and MPS.

Plate 3-39 Cytoplasmic Granules Associated with Birman Cat Anomaly

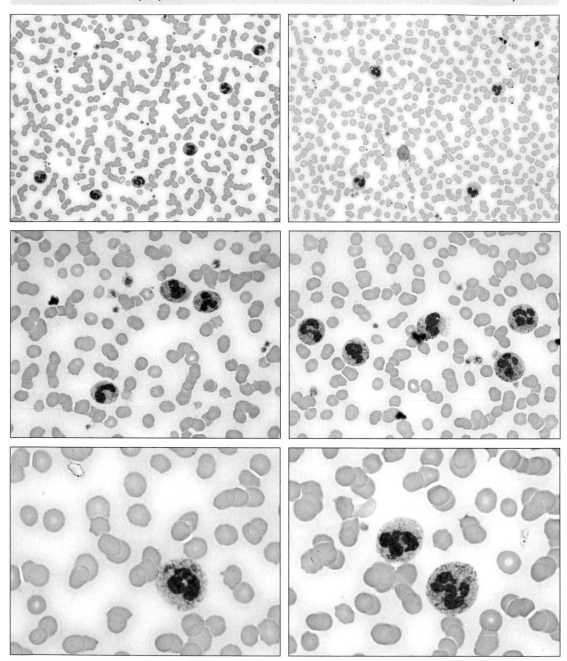

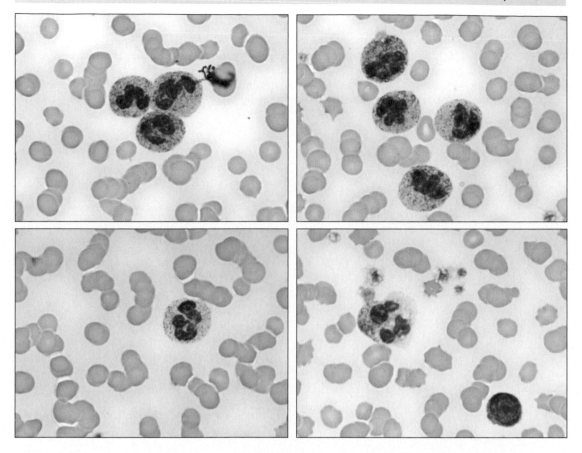

A, Toxic granulation **B,** Mucopolysaccharidosis **C,** Birman Cat Anomaly
D, Chédiak-Higashi Syndrome **E,** Primary neutrophil granules

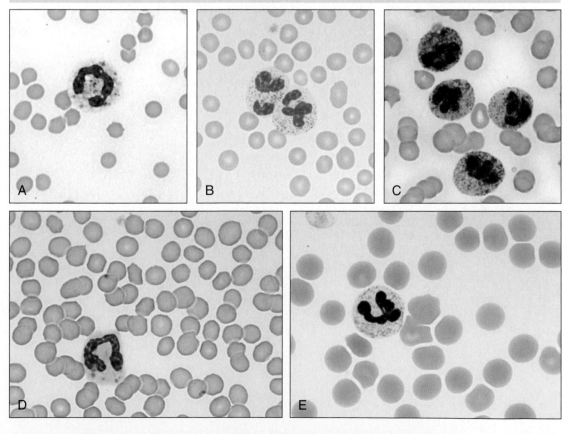

GM Gangliosidosis

DISTINCTIVE FEATURES: GM gangliosidosis, which is an uncommon inherited lysosomal storage disorder of dogs and cats, occurs in two forms. In GM_1 gangliosidosis, small, punctate, clear cytoplasmic vacuoles are found in lymphocytes. In GM_2 gangliosidosis, azurophilic granules are found in the cytoplasm of lymphocytes, and dark purple granules are found in neutrophils.

Plate 3-40   Cytoplasmic Vacuoles Associated with GM₁ Gangliosidosis

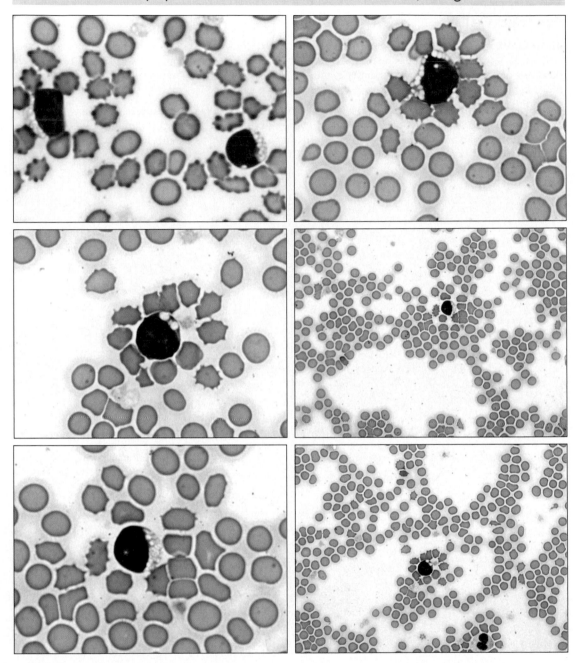

White Blood Cell Artifacts

Pyknotic Cells

DISTINCTIVE FEATURES: Pyknosis occurs in senescent (old) leukocytes and results from preprogrammed cell death (apoptosis). With pyknosis, the nucleus becomes dense and compact and begins to fragment (karyorrhexis) resulting in spheres of dark-staining nuclear chromatin. Therefore, pyknotic cells have an intact cytoplasmic membrane with one or more, variably sized, dense, round, dark nuclear fragments.

DIAGNOSTIC SIGNIFICANCE: The presence of pyknotic cells generally indicates a delay (hours) in making the blood smear after blood collection. Although pyknotic cells are often neutrophils because of their short life span and because they are typically the most numerous leukocyte, the identity of pyknotic cells cannot be determined. Preparation of blood smears as soon as possible after blood collection will help avoid such artifacts.

Plate 3-41   Pyknotic Cells

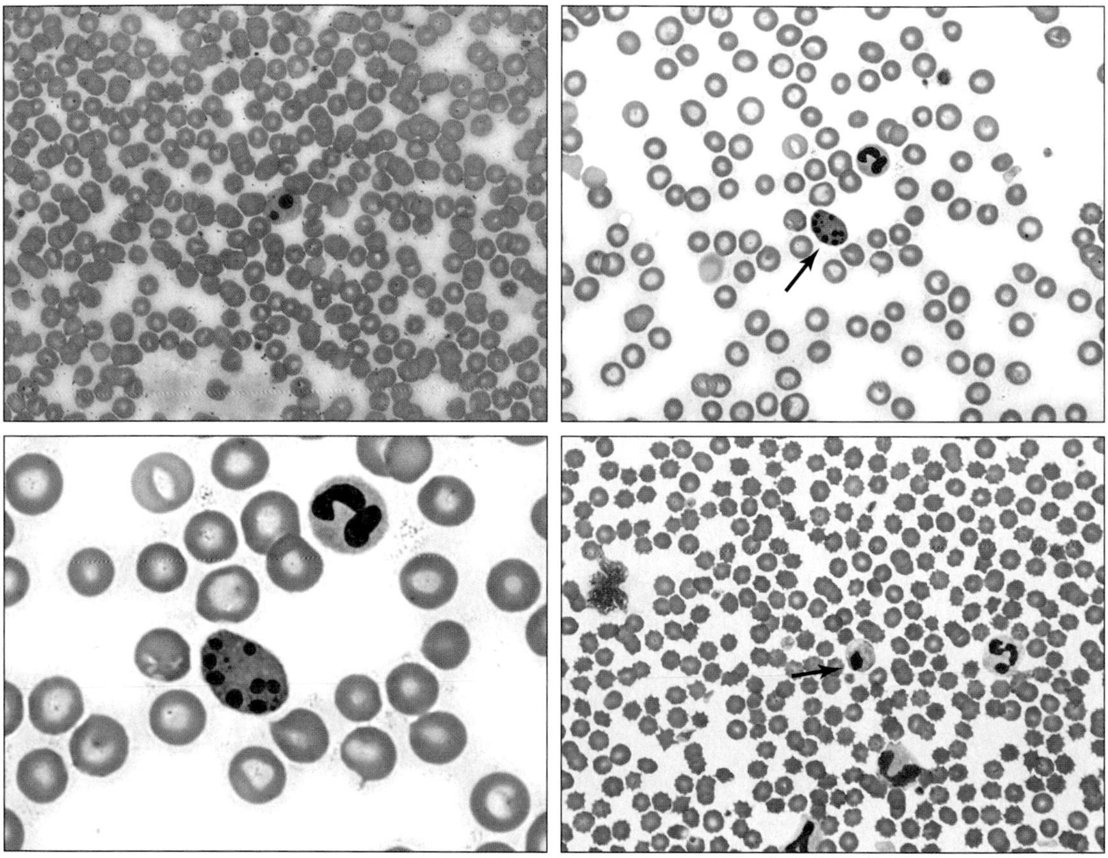

Plate 3-41 Pyknotic Cells *(con't)*

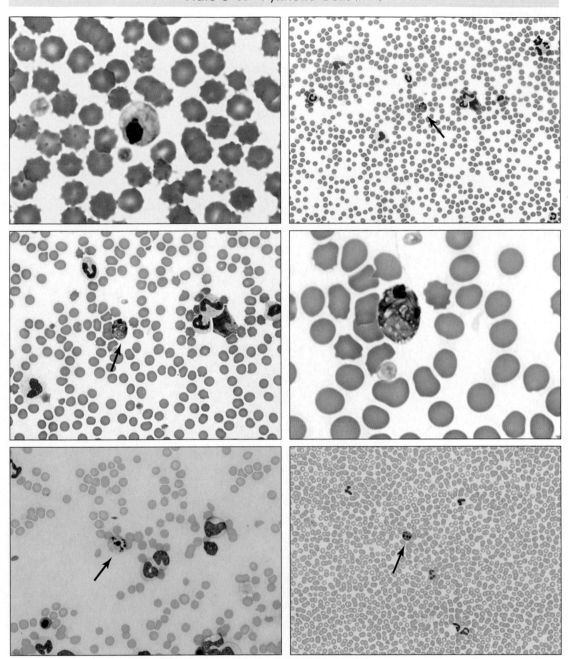

Basket or Smudge Cells

DISTINCTIVE FEATURES: Bare or free nuclei occur when WBCs rupture during blood smear preparation. The free nucleus may retain a similar appearance to the intact cell nucleus, or the nuclear chromatin may spread out and form an amorphous, netlike, eosinophilic structure (basket cell).

DIAGNOSTIC SIGNIFICANCE: Free nuclei and basket cells represent ruptured nucleated cells, and a few are commonly seen on many blood smears. Increased numbers may be seen with leukocytosis because of the increased number of leukocytes and increased chances of rupture. Also, conditions with high numbers of nucleated RBCs may increase the number of basket cells.

Plate 3-42 Basket/Smudge Cells

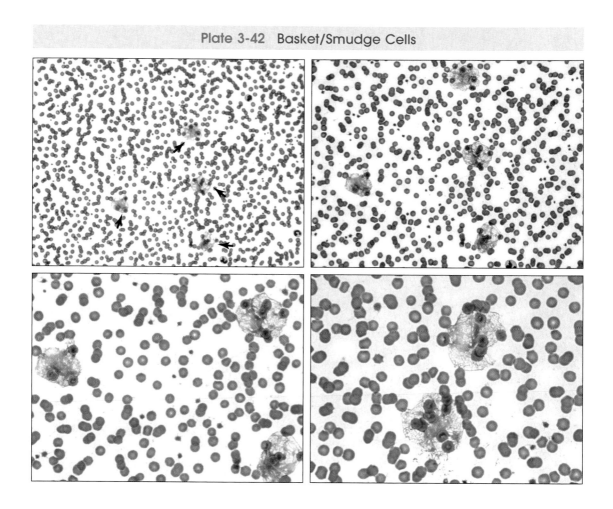

Plate 3-42   Basket/Smudge Cells *(con't)*

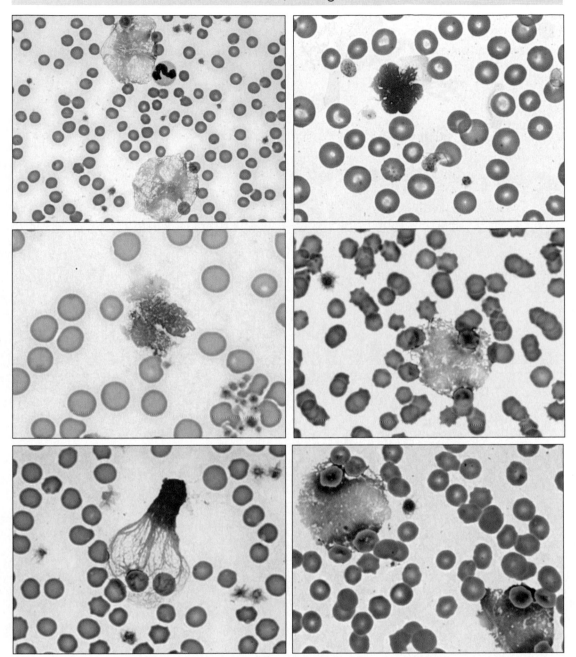

Platelet over White Blood Cell

DISTINCTIVE FEATURES: Occasionally platelets will overlie WBCs and may be readily identified by adjusting the fine focus of the microscope.

DIAGNOSTIC SIGNIFICANCE: Platelets over WBCs (or RBCs) are incidental findings of no clinical significance and must be distinguished from parasites or inclusions.

Plate 3-43   Platelets Overlying White Blood Cells

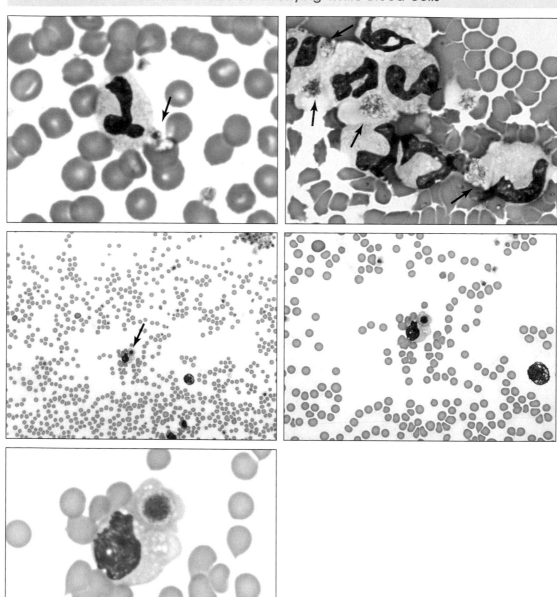

A, Döhle bodies **B,** Canine neutrophil with *Ehrlichia* morulae
C, Distemper inclusions **D,** Platelet over neutrophil

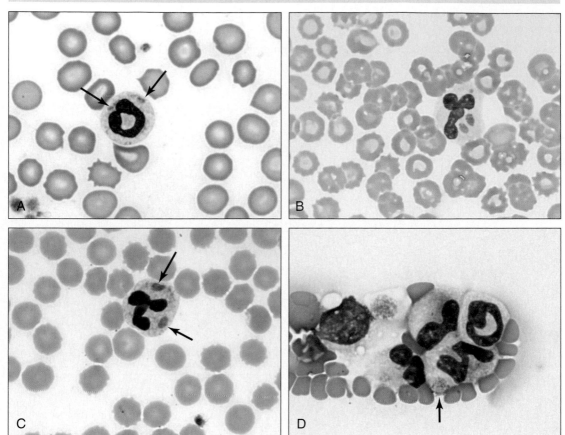

Changes Associated with Delayed Processing

DISTINCTIVE FEATURES: If blood smears are not made in a timely fashion, the cells age and degenerate. Neutrophil nuclei become poorly defined and appear to have smudged borders and homogenized chromatin.

DIAGNOSTIC SIGNIFICANCE: Recognize cellular aging changes associated with increased storage of blood prior to making smears.

Plate 3-44   Neutrophils Affected by Delayed Blood Smear Preparation

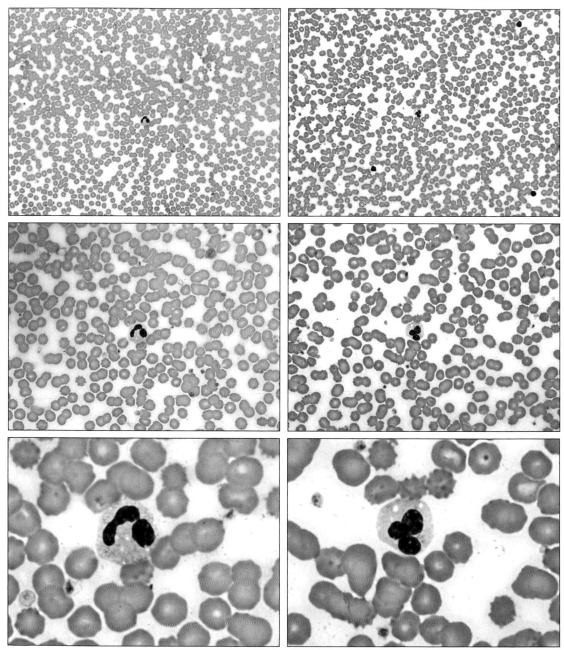

Plate 3-44   Neutrophils Affected by Delayed Blood Smear Preparation *(con't)*

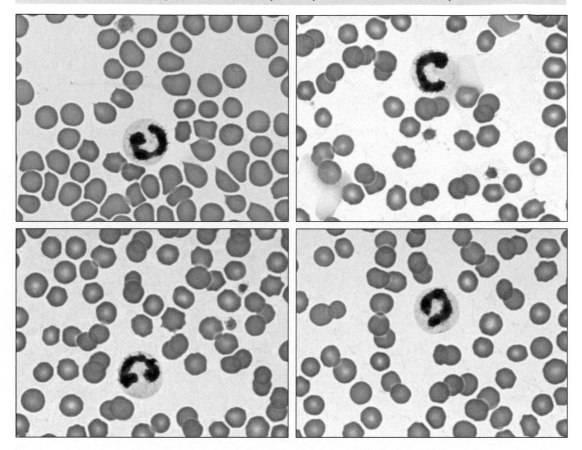

Understained Smears

DISTINCTIVE FEATURES: Understained smears have pale-staining leukocytes with ill-defined nuclear features.

DIAGNOSTIC SIGNIFICANCE: Recognize smears that are understained, and avoid false identification of inclusions and intracellular organisms.

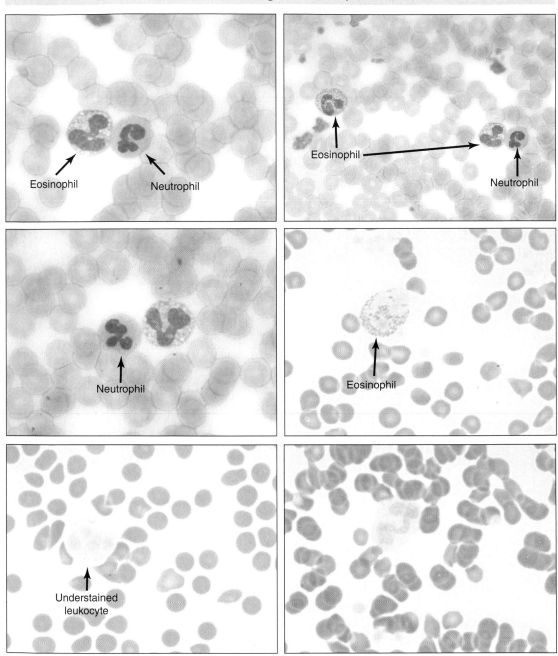

Plate 3-45 Understained Blood Films and Subsequent Poor Staining of Leukocytes

Plate 3-45 Understained Blood Films and Subsequent
Poor Staining of Leukocytes *(con't)*

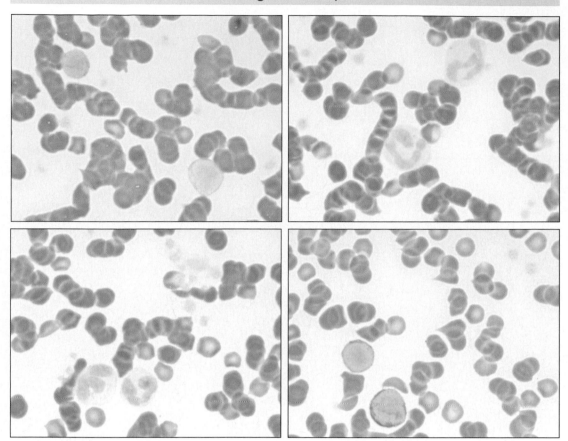

SECTION 4: PLATELETS

Normal Morphology

DISTINCTIVE FEATURES: Platelets are cytoplasmic fragments that form from bone marrow megakaryocytes (platelet progenitors) and are the smallest formed element in peripheral blood. As platelets are cytoplasmic fragments, they have no nucleus and generally appear as light blue to light pink, round to oval structures, with few to many small reddish granules.

DIAGNOSTIC SIGNIFICANCE: One of the most important functions of platelets is the role they play in hemostasis, requiring both adequate platelet numbers and normal platelet function. Blood smear review is important in assessing the number of platelets as well as evaluation of platelet size, shape, and granularity. Canine and feline blood smears should have between 7 and 35 platelets on the average of ten 100× oil objective fields in the monolayer to be considered adequate. Feline platelets tend to become activated easily during collection, handling of the blood sample, or both; thus, feline platelets often clump, resulting in falsely decreased platelet counts and estimates.

Plate 4-1   Normal Platelets

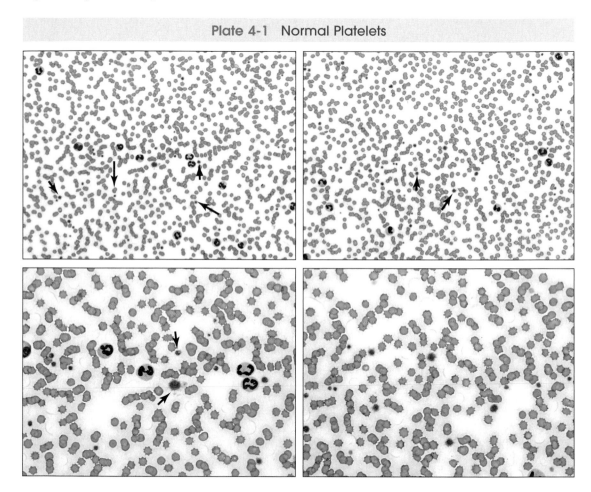

Plate 4-1 Normal Platelets *(con't)*

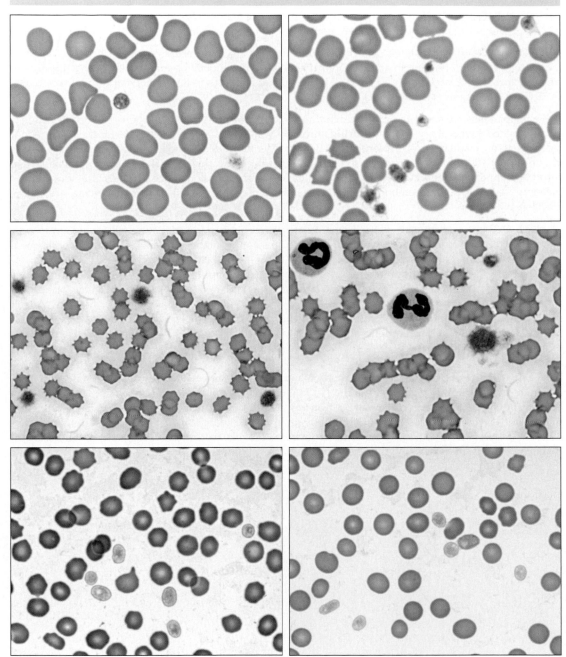

Thrombocytopenia

DISTINCTIVE FEATURES: Thrombocytopenia is the absence of platelet clumps and less than seven platelets per oil power field (100× objective) on an average for 10 or more fields.

DIAGNOSTIC SIGNIFICANCE: Be sure that platelet clumps are not present, as this will falsely decrease the platelet estimate, leading to an erroneous diagnosis of thrombocytopenia. If platelet clumps are not present, then each platelet seen on average in the 100× (oil objective) field equals approximately 15,000 to 20,000 platelets per microliter (µL).

Feline platelets are small and often similar in size to erythrocytes and may not be counted as platelets by automated hematology analyzers. Mild thrombocytopenia (100,000 to 200,000 platelets/µL) is not recognized on evaluation of a blood film. Only moderate and marked thrombocytopenias (platelet counts below 100,000/µL) are recognized. This is not a problem, since increased bleeding secondary to thrombocytopenia alone does not occur until platelet numbers are below 50,000/µL, and spontaneous bleeding secondary to thrombocytopenia alone does not occur until platelet numbers are below 25,000/µL.

NEXT STEPS: If platelet clumps have been ruled out and a true thrombocytopenia is evident, investigation for the underlying pathologic mechanisms for thrombocytopenia should be performed. Three main mechanisms of thrombocytopenia occur secondary to many different etiologies: (1) decreased platelet production (certain drugs and toxins, immune-mediated destruction of platelets, megakaryocytes, or both; neoplasia of the bone marrow); (2) decreased platelet survival (blood loss, disseminated intravascular coagulation [DIC], immune-mediated destruction); and (3) platelet sequestration (secondary to enlarged spleen). If a cause cannot be established, bone marrow cytology is often very helpful in determining if disease of the marrow is the cause of persistent, unexplained thrombocytopenia).

When evidence of clinical bleeding is present, and platelet numbers and coagulation times (prothrombin time [PT], partial thromboplastin time [PTT]) are normal, then investigation into platelet function defects should be considered with platelet function tests. Diseases resulting in altered platelet function may be both hereditary (Basset Hound thrombopathia, Chédiak-Higashi syndrome, cyclic hematopoiesis in Grey Collies, Glanzmann's thrombasthenia of Great Pyrenees and Otterhounds), and acquired (drugs, toxins, infections, neoplasia, hyperglobulinemia).

Plate 4-2   Thrombocytopenia

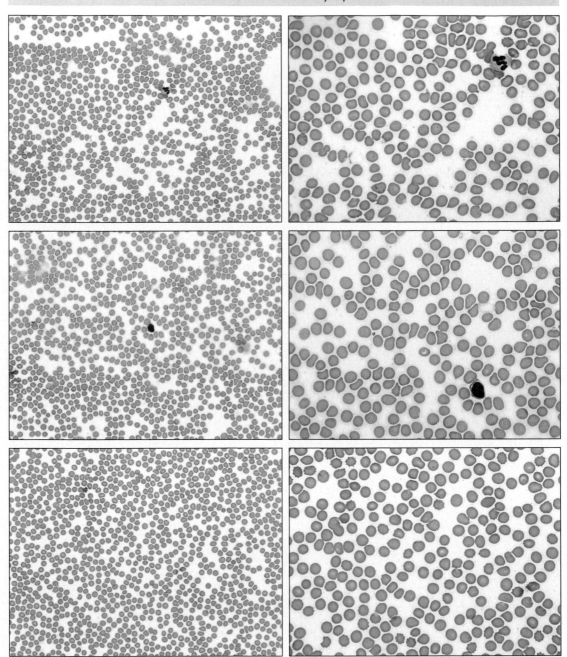

Plate 4-2 Thrombocytopenia *(con't)*

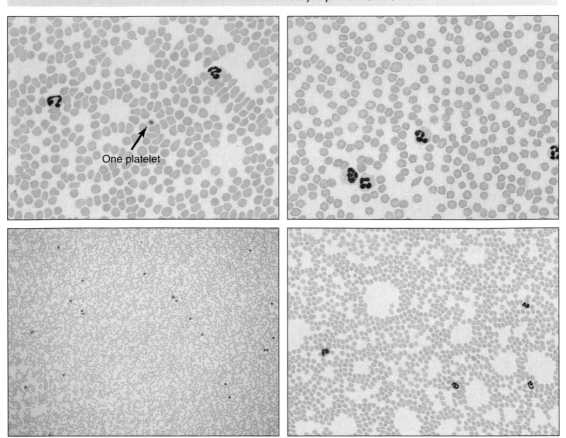

One platelet

Artifactual thrombocytopenia. **A,** Monolayer, devoid of platelets
B, Feathered edge large platelet clumps

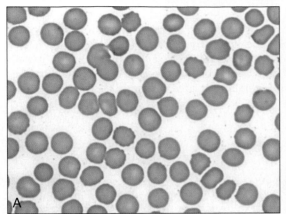

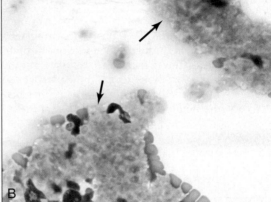

Thrombocytosis

DISTINCTIVE FEATURES: Greater than 35 platelets per oil power field (100×) objective on an average of 10 or more fields.

DIAGNOSTIC SIGNIFICANCE: Physiologic thrombocytosis (increased platelet production) is the most common cause of thrombocytosis, occurring secondary to a reactive process (i.e., inflammation, iron deficiency anemia in dogs, rebound from thrombocytopenia, chronic blood loss anemia), with platelet counts typically fewer than 1,000,000 platelets/μL (<60 platelets per oil power field [100× objective] on an average of 10 or more fields). If the platelet count is persistently greater than 1,000,000 platelets/μL, then essential thrombocythemia and acute megakaryocytic leukemia should be considered, both of which are very rare hemic neoplasms of dogs and cats.

Plate 4-3   Thrombocytosis

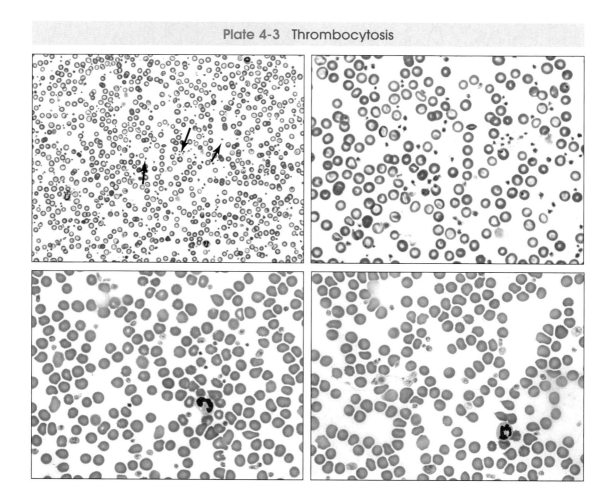

Plate 4-3 Thrombocytosis *(con't)*

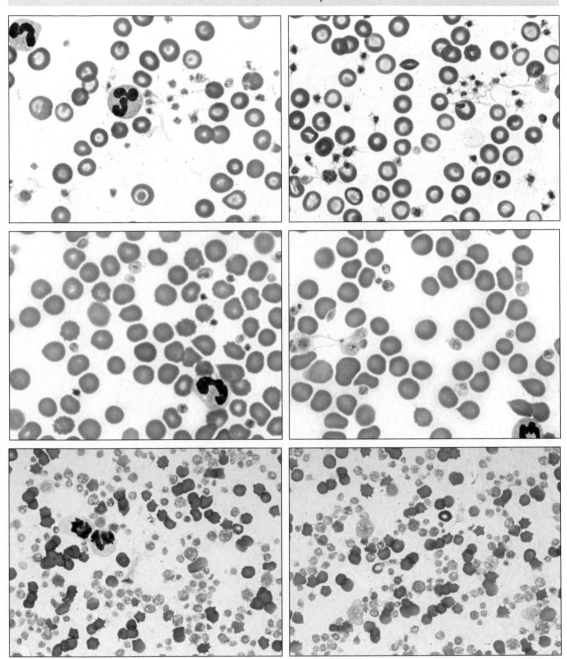

Platelet Clumps

DISTINCTIVE FEATURES: Platelet clumps may appear as groups of distinct platelets, but degranulated platelet clumps may appear as blue blobs, which are difficult to recognize as platelet clumps. Because of their large size, platelet clumps may be concentrated on the feathered edge, but smaller clumps may also be present in the monolayer.

DIAGNOSTIC SIGNIFICANCE: Platelet clumping is typically an artifact secondary to platelet activation during collection, handling of peripheral blood, or both. Platelet clumping is a common problem in cats. Platelet clumps result in platelet counts (manual and machine generated) being falsely decreased, and severe clumping may result in the platelet count being falsely reported as thrombocytopenia (pseudo-thrombocytopenia). Also, some conditions cause platelets to be hyperactive, so they are more prone to being activated, resulting in platelet clumps. If many platelet clumps are present in a patient that has a low platelet count, it should be considered pseudothrombocytopenia. When many platelet clumps are present, the patient is considered to have sufficient numbers of platelets to not spontaneously bleed from thrombocytopenia alone, regardless of the platelet count generated by the hematology analyzer.

Plate 4-4   Platelet Clumps

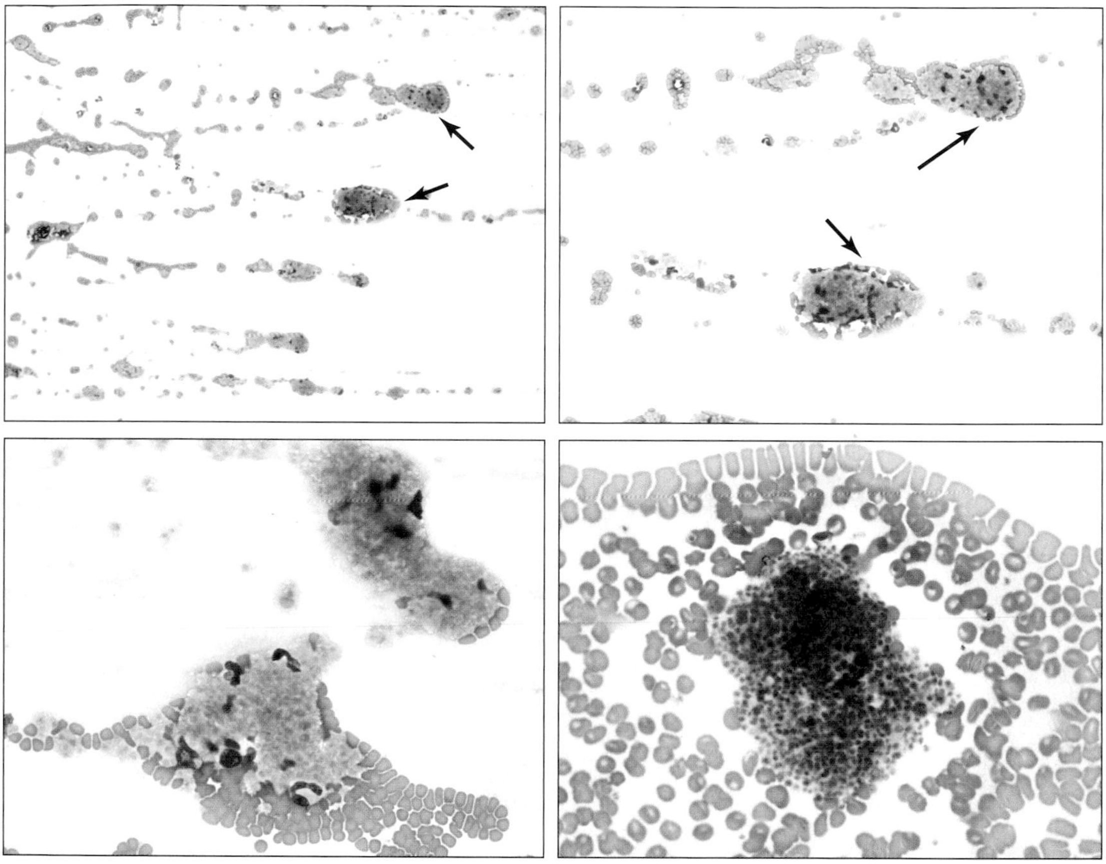

Plate 4-4 Platelet Clumps (con't)

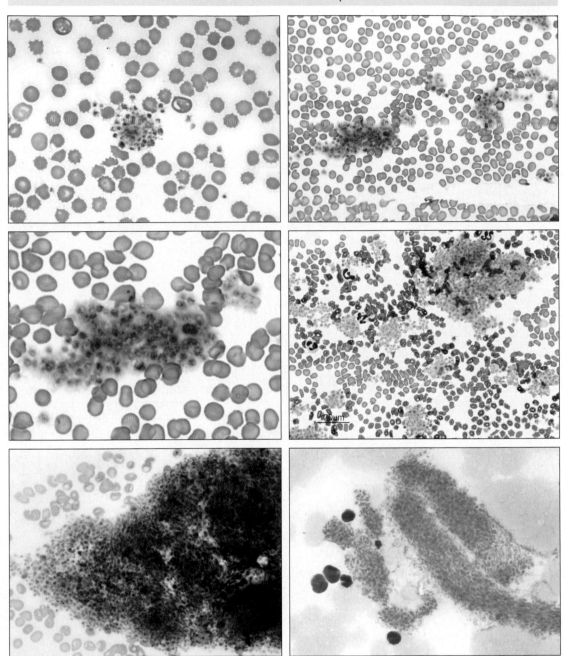

Activated Platelets

DISTINCTIVE FEATURES: Activated platelets have thin cytoplasmic projections. The platelet granules may become condensed in the center of the platelet and should not be mistaken for a nucleus. Also, activated platelets may degranulate, and few or no reddish intracytoplasmic granules may be present. Degranulated platelet clumps may appear as bluish blobs, which are difficult to recognize as platelet clumps.

DIAGNOSTIC SIGNIFICANCE: Platelet activation is typically an artifact that occurs during collection, and/or handling of peripheral blood, or both. Feline platelets activate easily, and activated platelets and platelet clumps are common findings. Make sure not to confuse activated platelets with infectious agents such as trypanosomes and sphirochetes.

Plate 4-5   Activated Platelets

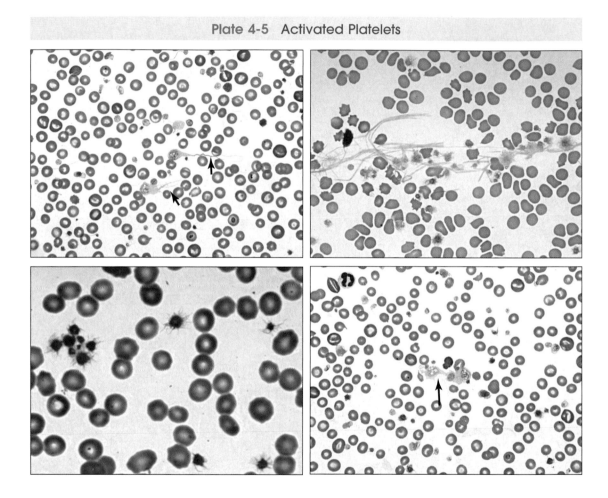

Plate 4-5 Activated Platelets *(con't)*

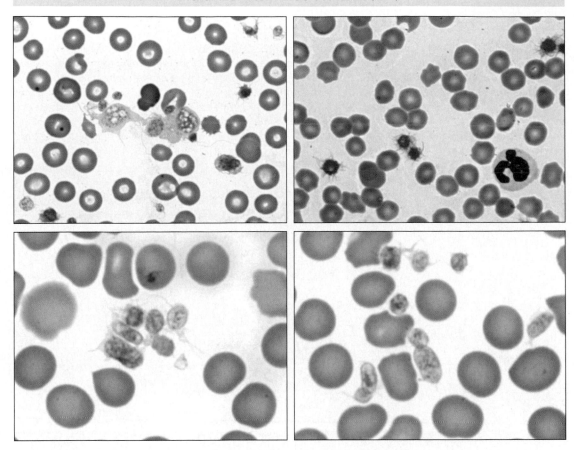

Make sure not to confuse activated platelets with infectious organisms such as trypanosomes and spirochetes. **A,** Trypanosoma spp. **B,** Spirochetes spp. **C,** Activated platelets

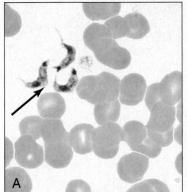
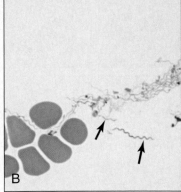
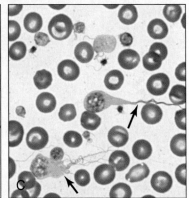

Macroplatelets (Megaplatelets)

DISTINCTIVE FEATURES: Platelets that are greater than 5 μm in diameter (as large as or larger than feline red blood cells [RBCs]).

DIAGNOSTIC SIGNIFICANCE: Low numbers of megaplatelets may be seen on peripheral blood smears from normal cats. Increased numbers of megaplatelets in thrombocytopenic dogs suggests increased thrombopoiesis; however, this also may be seen in myeloproliferative and myelodysplastic disorders. Megaplatelets may also be seen on blood smears from healthy animals with hereditary platelet function defects. Some Cavalier King Charles Spaniels may have congenital macrothrombocytopenia, which is a benign inherited giant platelet disorder. These patients may be thrombocytopenic and have megaplatelets. The platelets of these dogs function normally, and despite low numbers of platelets, bleeding abnormalities are absent, as the platelet mass is normal.

Plate 4-6   Macroplatelets

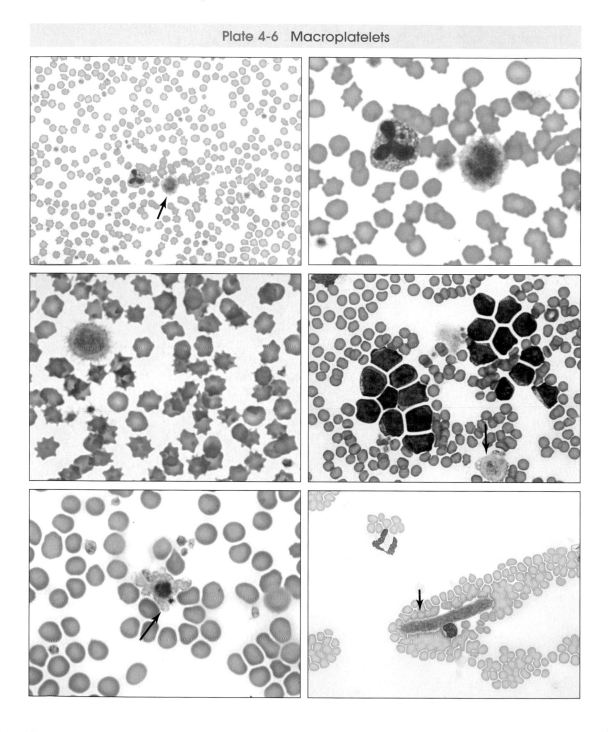

Plate 4-6   Macroplatelets *(con't)*

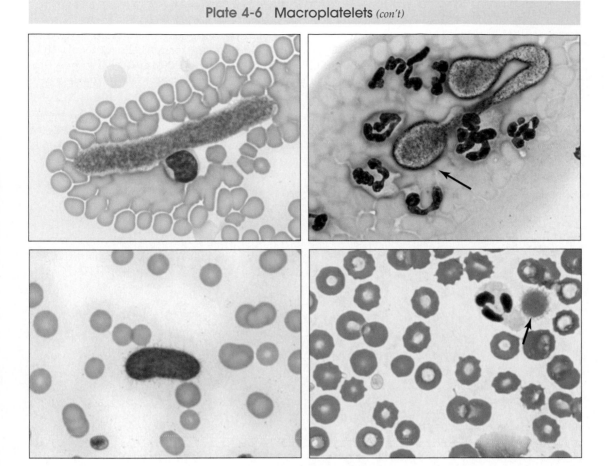

Megakaryocytes

DISTINCTIVE FEATURES: Megakaryocytes are bone marrow platelet progenitors, which undergo endomitosis rather than mitosis and cell division. Megakaryocytes are extremely large cells (generally 50 to 150 μm), which have a single nucleus with multiple lobes (2–16). The cytoplasm is blue to pink and moderate to abundant, both dependent on the maturity of the cell. Megakaryocytes also contain few to many reddish intracytoplasmic granules.

DIAGNOSTIC SIGNIFICANCE: Megakaryocytes are an extremely rare finding on peripheral blood smears from normal animals. If present, secondary to their large size, megakaryocytes are usually found at the feathered edge. Megakaryocytes may be observed in the peripheral blood with megakaryocytic leukemia (very rare), which may be associated with either thrombocytosis or thrombocytopenia and morphologically abnormal platelets.

Plate 4-7   Megakaryocytes

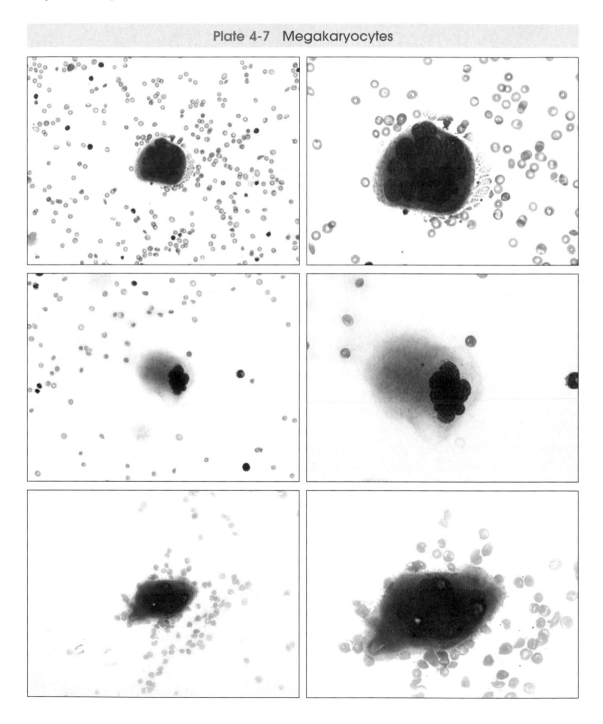

Plate 4-7 Megakaryocytes *(con't)*

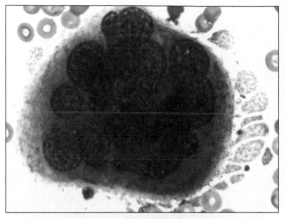
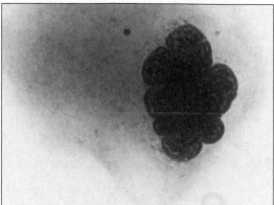
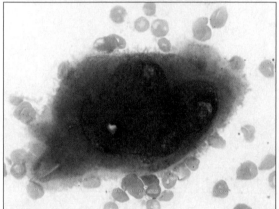
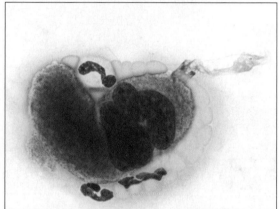

Parasites

Anaplasma platys (formerly *Erhlichia platys*)

DISTINCTIVE FEATURES: *Anaplasma platys* (formerly *Ehrlichia platys*) is a tickborne intracellular bacterium that infects platelets, resulting in infectious cyclic thrombocytopenia in dogs. The organisms appear as a blue-black cluster within platelets.

DIAGNOSTIC SIGNIFICANCE: Finding intracellular *Anaplasma platys* organisms in the cytoplasm of canine platelets is diagnostic. Infection is associated with thrombocytopenia. If diagnosed, assessment for other tickborne diseases is advised to rule out co-infection.

Plate 4-8   *Anaplasma platys*

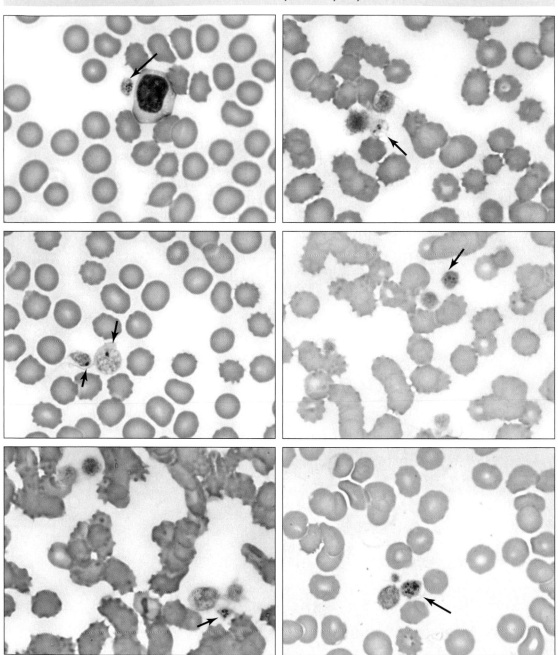

Plate 4-8   *Anaplasma platys* (con't)

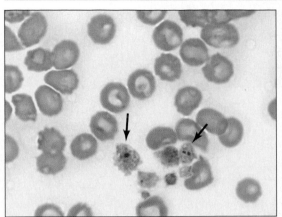
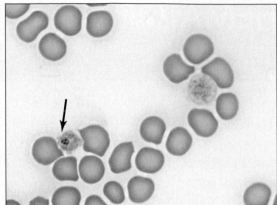
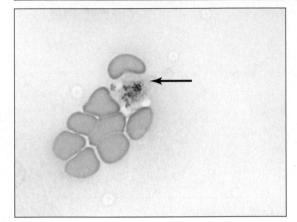

SECTION 5:
HEMATOPOIETIC NEOPLASIA

Overview

Leukemia is defined as a clonal proliferation of neoplastic cells originating in bone marrow. Leukemia of every peripheral blood cell type has been identified in dogs and cats. Lymphoid leukemia (both acute and chronic forms) is common in dogs and cats, whereas leukemias of the other cell lines are quite uncommon. Diagnosis of leukemia is based on clinical presentation (clinical signs and physical examination), and laboratory data, including complete blood count (CBC) and serum chemistry analysis. The findings of large numbers of neoplastic cells on CBC and blood smear microscopic evaluation are one important part of the diagnosis and classification of the various leukemias. Definitive diagnosis may often require bone marrow evaluation.

Many different leukemia classification schemes have been proposed and utilized. Various schemes are based on a mix of information such as clinical behavior (response to therapy, survival time), cellular morphology (microscopic evaluation of the neoplastic cells), histopathology (neoplastic pattern on tissue biopsy), topography (extent of neoplastic involvement), phenotype (genetic expression), and genotype (genetic characteristics and aberrations) of the neoplastic cell population.

Although blood smear evaluation remains an important part of diagnosis and classification of leukemias, it is important to recognize that morphology alone is not sufficient to classify various leukemias. This is especially true with the acute forms of leukemia, as blasts of various lineages may appear morphologically identical.

Two large categories of leukemia exist: (1) lymphoid leukemias and (2) myeloid (nonlymphoid) leukemias, with acute and chronic forms of each category. Acute leukemias are composed of blast cells. This type of leukemia manifests acutely and is aggressive, often associated with large numbers of circulating blasts, peripheral blood cytopenias, occasional secondary organ infiltration, and a poorer prognosis compared with that for chronic leukemias.

With regard to acute leukemias, identification of the lineage of the blast cell population may be difficult, especially if it is solely based on light-microscopic morphologic features with routine hematologic stains. Blast cells may sometimes have distinct features to suggest phenotype; however, most appear similar microscopically, and further tests are needed to identify ontogeny. Such tests aiding in differentiation may include cytochemical staining using enzymes and immunocytochemistry or flow cytometry, which utilize labeled antibodies targeted against specified antigens found in various cell lines (immunophenotyping). Furthermore, clonality tests are available for identifying lymphoid leukemias, to assess whether a population of lymphoid cells are clonal in origin (suggestive of neoplasia) or nonclonal (suggestive of inflammation or reactivity). Identification of genetic abnormalities (cytogenetics) is increasingly playing a role in the classification of leukemias in veterinary medicine.

In contrast to acute leukemias, chronic leukemias develop more slowly, are not often associated with cytopenias until the late stage of disease, often do not have organ involvement, and are associated with a more favorable prognosis. The neoplastic cell population in chronic leukemias comprises mature, well-differentiated cells that are often morphologically identical to normal blood leukocytes. Thus, the mature morphology of the neoplastic cells may make it very difficult to distinguish leukemia from inflammatory processes. Differentiation is based on ruling out sources of infection, inflammation, or immunostimulation and continued monitoring of the CBC over time to document the persistence, and increasing numbers, of one type of leukocyte.

A brief overview of the different types of leukemias in dogs and cats is presented in this chapter, with an emphasis on morphologic features.

Lymphoid Leukemia

Acute Lymphoblastic Leukemia

DISTINCTIVE FEATURES: Acute lymphoblastic leukemia (ALL) is a neoplastic proliferation of lymphoblasts and may be either B-cell or T-cell phenotype. Lymphoblasts are large cells, often 1.5 to 2 times the diameter of neutrophils. Lymphoblasts contain slight to moderate amounts of basophilic cytoplasm, a round to oval eccentrically placed nucleus, stippled to slightly coarse nuclear chromatin, and often either faint or, more commonly, prominent nucleoli. Nucleoli are typically singular, but occasionally, two nucleoli may be present.

DIAGNOSTIC SIGNIFICANCE: Lymphoblasts are rarely seen in the peripheral blood of normal dogs and cats. Occasional lymphoblasts may be seen in peripheral blood with strong immune stimulation. Low to high numbers of lymphoblasts may be seen in peripheral blood with lymphoblastic leukemia. Classic

CBC findings with ALL include large numbers of circulating blasts and, often, one or multiple cytopenias.

NEXT STEPS: Light microscopy alone cannot reliably distinguish T-cell ALL from B-cell ALL, nor can it reliably distinguish lymphoblasts from myeloblasts or monoblasts. Other methods such as immunocytochemistry and flow cytometry are needed to define exact phenotype. B-cell leukemia is associated with a more favorable prognosis compared with T-cell leukemia.

Low to occasional to moderate numbers of circulating lymphoblasts may be seen with stage V lymphoma, indicating neoplastic seeding of bone marrow and the subsequent leukemic phase. Distinguishing stage V lymphoma from late stage lymphoid leukemia may be difficult. Determining the location of the bulk of neoplastic involvement (marrow or blood versus solid tissue) may be used to distinguish the conditions.

Finding low to high numbers of blasts in peripheral blood warrants assessment for involvement of lymphoreticular organs for staging purposes.

Plate 5-1   Acute Lymphoblastic Leukemia

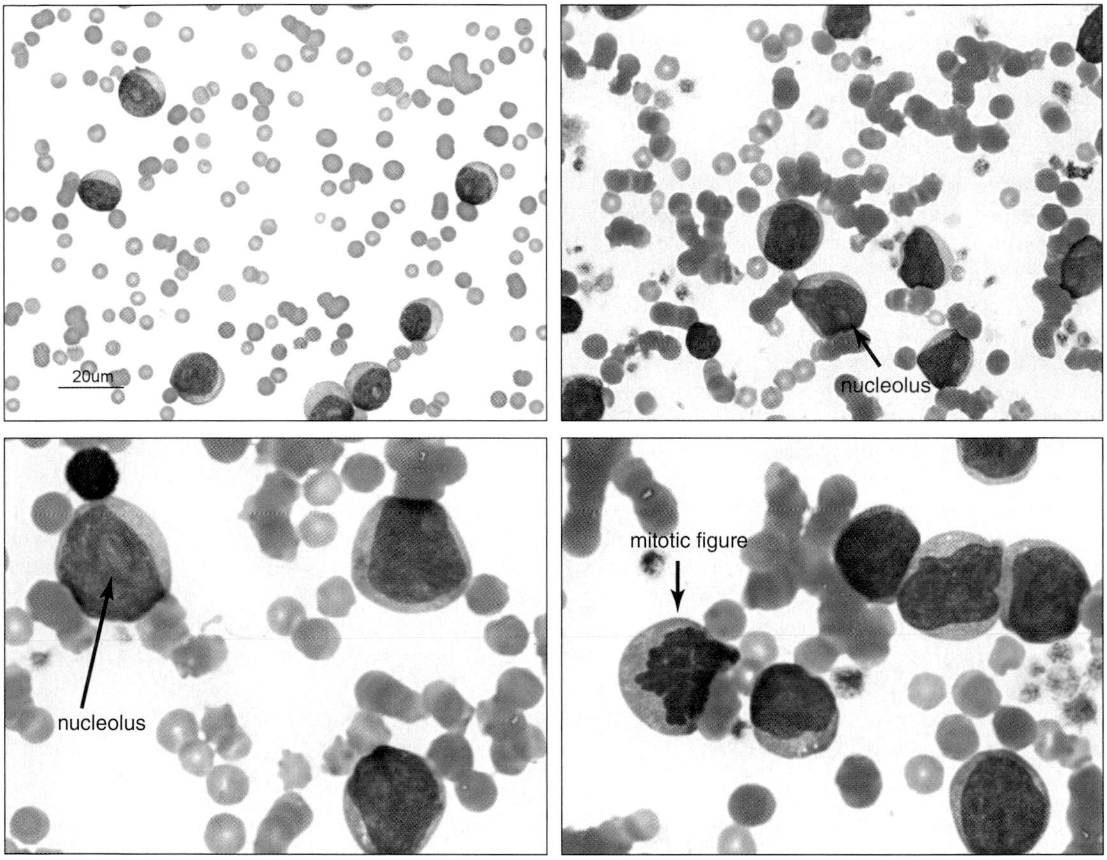

Plate 5-1   Acute Lymphoblastic Leukemia *(con't)*

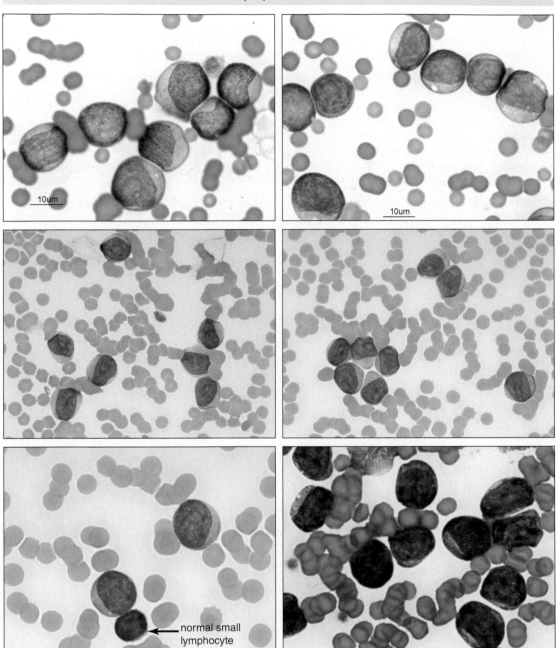

normal small lymphocyte

Chronic Lymphocytic Leukemia

DISTINCTIVE FEATURES: Chronic lymphocytic leukemia (CLL) is a neoplastic proliferation of small, mature lymphocytes. Morphology is identical to that of nonneoplastic mature lymphocytes. The lymphocytosis in CLL may be mild in early stages and marked in later stages. Cytopenias are uncommon and typically only seen when the neoplastic cells are present in very high numbers.

DIAGNOSTIC SIGNIFICANCE: CLL is most often a leukemia found in older dogs and cats. When a mild to moderate lymphocytosis is present, distinguishing it from a reactive population of lymphocytes secondary to immunostimulation may be difficult and relies on monitoring of the CBC over time (persistent lymphocytosis, often with a slowly progressive increase in numbers). Immunophenotypic analysis and documentation of a monoclonal population may also lend support to the diagnosis of leukemia. In addition, clonality testing is also available to help identify clonal populations of lymphocytes. It is important to recognize that clonality by itself is not diagnostic of neoplasia. As an example, clonal populations of T lymphocytes have been identified in dogs with chronic ehrlichiosis.

NEXT STEPS: As for ALL, distinguishing between B-cell and T-cell phenotypes is not possible with light microscopy alone, and further techniques are required. When CLL is diagnosed, assessment for involvement of the lymphoreticular organs is advised to further stage the disease.

A diagnosis of CLL warrants monitoring of the CBC, despite treatment, as evolution into a blast crisis may occur, culminating in an acute leukemia.

Plate 5-2   Chronic Lymphocytic Leukemia

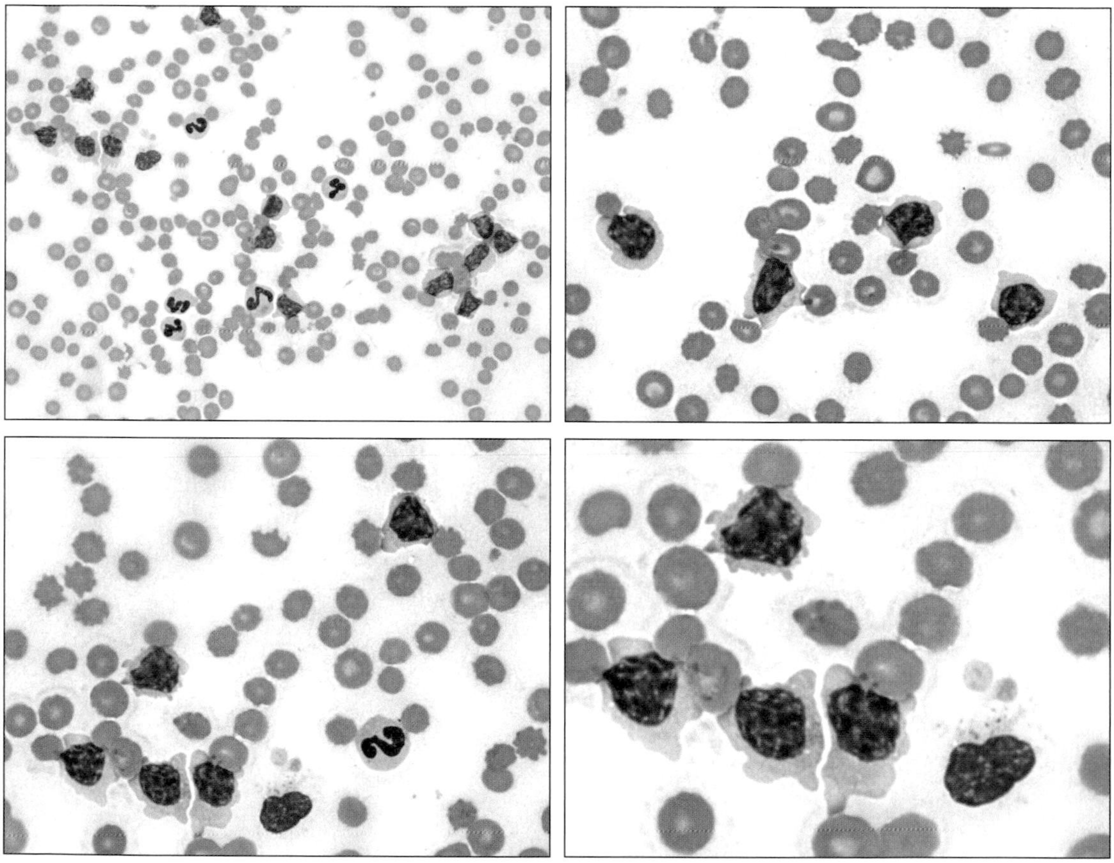

Plate 5-2 Chronic Lymphocytic Leukemia *(con't)*

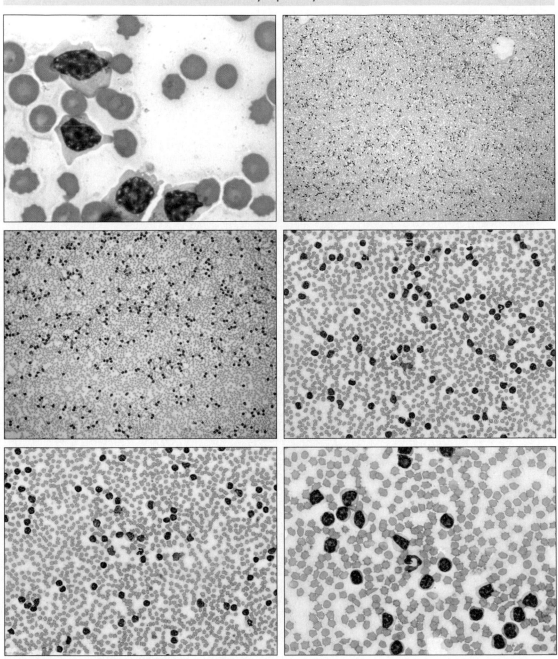

T-Cell Large Granular Lymphocytic Leukemia

DISTINCTIVE FEATURES: T-cell large granular lymphocytic leukemia (T-cell LGL leukemia) is composed of large, immature T lymphocytes, with variable numbers of round to irregular, variably sized, magenta-staining cytoplasmic granules.

DIAGNOSTIC SIGNIFICANCE: Low numbers of nonneoplastic circulating granular lymphocytes may be seen in dogs and cats secondary to immunostimulation. In particular, low to moderate numbers of granular lymphocytes may be seen in dogs, with or without a mild lymphocytosis and with ehrlichiosis. Thus, as with CLL, ruling out etiologies of immunostimulation and monitoring of the CBC over time are needed to help confirm a leukemic process.

> **NEXT STEPS:** As for all of the lymphoid leukemias, assessment for lymphoreticular organ infiltration is suggested for staging. Although commonly referred to as *lymphocytic leukemia of granular lympho-cytes*, in dogs, this disorder actually arises in the spleen rather than in bone marrow.

Plate 5-3   T-Cell Large Granular Lymphocytic Leukemia

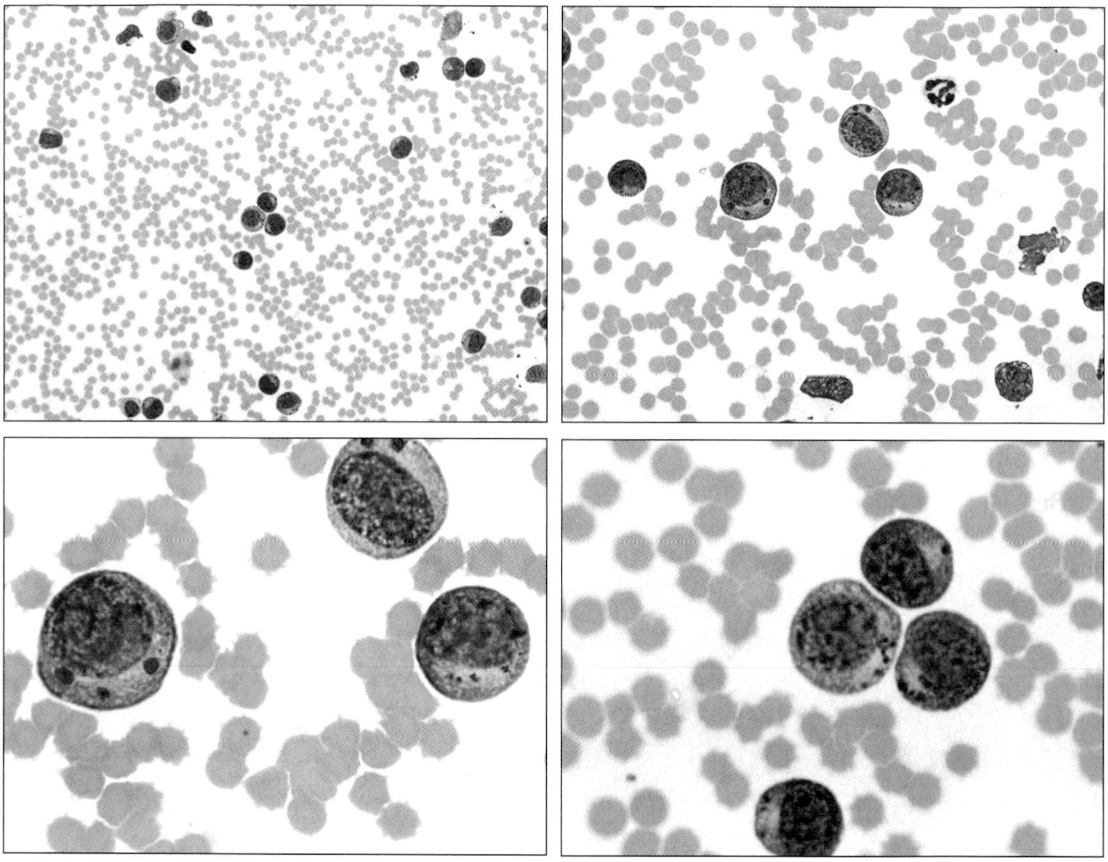

Plate 5-3   T-Cell Large Granular Lymphocytic Leukemia *(con't)*

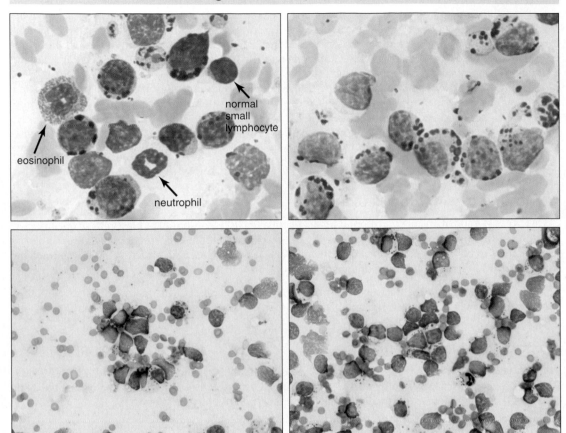

Acute Myeloid Leukemia

Acute myeloid leukemia (AML) is a group of acute leukemias composed of blast cells of one, or more than one, of the myeloid cell lines: granulocytic (neutrophils, eosinophils, basophils); monocytic; erythroid and megakaryocytic. Finding 20% or more blasts in blood or bone marrow is useful in diagnosis. In overt AML, blasts are present in blood and bone marrow in very high numbers, with cytopenias and possible lymphoreticular organ infiltration.

As with all acute leukemias, lineage is best determined through a combination of light-microscopic evaluation and assessment of phenotype by using cytochemical stains or immunophenotyping by flow cytometry.

AML must be distinguished from myelodysplastic syndromes (MDS), especially with feline leukemia virus (FeLV)–induced MDS in cats. Dysplastic changes may be seen with AML but are much more common in MDS; the presence of dysplasia warrants FeLV testing in cats and careful monitoring of the CBC, as MDS may progress to AML.

Acute Undifferentiated Leukemia

DISTINCTIVE FEATURES: Acute undifferentiated leukemia (AUL) is composed of blast cells of uncharacterized lineage (lymphoid or myeloid), where the cells lack any defining morphologic features and may have features of blasts of various lineages. The cells also lack cytochemical, structural, and immunologic markers to aid in determination of ontogeny.

AUL is diagnosed on the basis of the presence of greater than 20% of nucleated cells in blood or bone marrow constituting blast. Indeed, blasts are often in very high numbers both in blood and bone marrow.

Acute Myeloblastic Leukemia

DISTINCTIVE FEATURES: The three subtypes of acute myeloblastic leukemia are AML-M0, AML-M1, AML-M2, which are categorized by the degree of maturation and cellular differentiation of the neoplastic cells performed by microscopic evaluation and immunophenotypic assessment.

All three subcategories consist of 20% or more myeloblasts in blood, bone marrow, or both (usually large numbers of blasts are present, often approaching 100% of all nucleated cells).

Myeloblasts are difficult to distinguish from primitive blasts of other hematopoietic cell lines, and sometimes even from lymphoblasts. Myeloblasts are about the same size, or slightly smaller than, promyelocytes. They have round to oval, centrally located nuclei, which contain finely stippled chromatin and one to several visible nucleoli. A small to moderate amount of moderately basophilic cytoplasm is present and, at the later blast stage, may contain a few to several magenta-staining granules. Very immature myeloblasts may lack granules altogether.

DIAGNOSTIC SIGNIFICANCE: It is extremely rare to see myeloblasts in peripheral blood smears from healthy dogs and cats. Finding a myeloblast in a peripheral blood smear always raises the concern of granulocytic leukemia (although it must be kept in mind that it is difficult, if not impossible, to reliably distinguish myeloblasts from lymphoblasts on the basis of morphology alone). However, rarely, a myeloblast may be seen in peripheral blood with severe inflammation, as part of an orderly left shift with toxic change. In addition, rare immature hematopoietic precursors may be found in peripheral blood secondary to toxic or hypoxic damage to bone marrow.

NEXT STEPS: The persistent (progressive) presence of a few to large numbers of blasts in blood warrants bone marrow examination. Serial CBC and bone marrow examinations may be needed for diagnosis, especially if the leukemia is in an early stage (low numbers of blasts).

Acute Promyelocytic Leukemia

DISTINCTIVE FEATURES: Acute promyelocytic leukemia (AML-M3) is an extremely uncommon leukemia in animals. Diagnosis is based on finding 20% or more atypical-appearing promyelocytes in peripheral blood, bone marrow, or both. Part of this count includes any identified myeloblasts as well.

The atypical-appearing promyelocytes may be hypergranular or poorly granular. Promyelocytes are of the same size or slightly larger than myeloblasts, with a slight increase in pale blue cytoplasm. When granules are present, they are azurophilic, small, and evenly distributed. Nuclei are round and slightly smaller than those of the myeloblast. Lacy to coarse chromatin is seen, with faint or visible nucleoli sometimes evident. Usually, nucleoli are fewer and more difficult to visualize compared with myeloblasts.

DIAGNOSTIC SIGNIFICANCE: AML-M3 is very uncommon and must be differentiated from a left shift caused by severe inflammation or infection and from myelodysplastic syndromes.

Acute Myelomonocytic Leukemia

DISTINCTIVE FEATURES: In acute myelomonocytic leukemia (AML-M4), the neoplastic cells are of mixed lineage, consisting of both immature myeloid cells and monocytic cells.

Bone marrow cytology is needed for diagnosis and is based on 20% or more of all nucleated bone marrow cells constituting myeloblasts, monoblasts, or promonocytes; 20% or more of all nucleated bone marrow cells having to be of monocytic lineage; and 20% or more of all nucleated bone marrow cells having to be of granulocytic lineage.

DIAGNOSTIC SIGNIFICANCE: Bone marrow cytology and cytochemical stains are helpful in distinguishing myeloid cells from cells of monocytic lineage when cell counts are performed.

Acute Monocytic Leukemia

DISTINCTIVE FEATURES: Acute monocytic leukemia (AML-M5) is diagnosed on the basis of 80% or more of all nucleated cells being of monocytic origin, with 20% or more of all nucleated cells consisting of myeloblasts, monoblasts, or promonocytes.

Of the two subtypes, AML-M5a is composed of more immature monocytic cells (acute monoblastic leukemia) and is more common in young animals. Here, monoblasts comprise 50% or more of monocytic cells. The second subtype, AML-M5b, is composed of more mature monocytic cells (acute monocytic leukemia) and is seen most often in older animals, and 50% or more of the monocytic cells are promonocytes.

Monoblasts are roundish cells with a moderate amount of basophilic cytoplasm and a round to oval nucleus that has an undulating outline. The nuclear chromatin ranges from stippled to stringy, and one or more nucleoli are visible. The irregular outline to the nuclear membrane is one of the more distinguishing features of the monoblast.

DIAGNOSTIC SIGNIFICANCE: Bone marrow cytology and cytochemical stains are helpful in the diagnosis of AML-M4.

Acute Erythroleukemia

DISTINCTIVE FEATURES: Acute erythroleukemia (AML-M6) is diagnosed by the presence of greater than 50% erythroid precursors in bone marrow. The two subtypes are AML-M6a, in which 20% or more of all bone marrow nucleated cells are myeloblasts. AML-M6b is characterized by 20% or more of all bone marrow nucleated cells consisting of myeloblasts and rubriblasts. The peripheral blood picture often contains large numbers of immature erythroid and myeloid cells, with dysplastic erythroid elements often seen in both subtypes.

Rubriblasts are round cells with dark blue cytoplasm and a roundish nucleus that is often centrally located but may be eccentrically placed. The nuclear chromatin is stippled, and one or more nucleoli are visible.

DIAGNOSTIC SIGNIFICANCE: AML-M6b is the subtype most commonly seen in animals, especially in FeLV-positive cats. AML-M6 must be differentiated from myelodysplastic syndromes, also frequently associated with FeLV infection in cats.

Rubriblasts are generally not seen in peripheral blood smears from healthy dogs and cats. Rubriblasts may rarely be seen with strongly regenerative anemia such as immune-mediated anemia in dogs and *Mycoplasma hemofelis* infection in cats. Also, rubriblasts may be seen in peripheral blood smears from animals with repopulating bone marrow after severe insult.

Plate 5-4   Acute Erythroleukemia

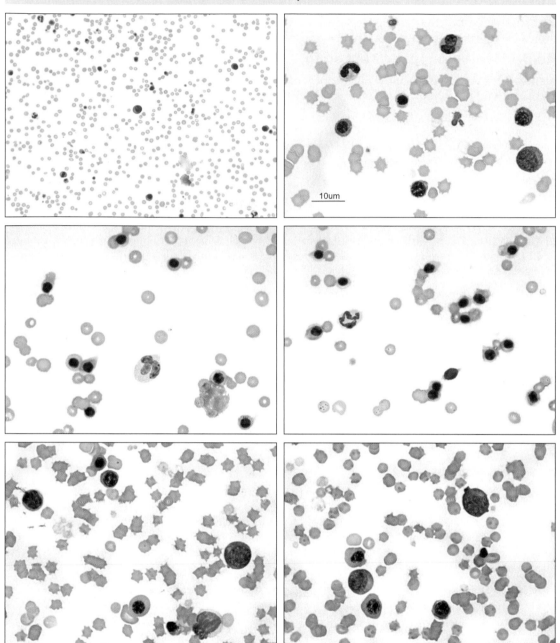

Plate 5-4 Acute Erythroleukemia *(con't)*

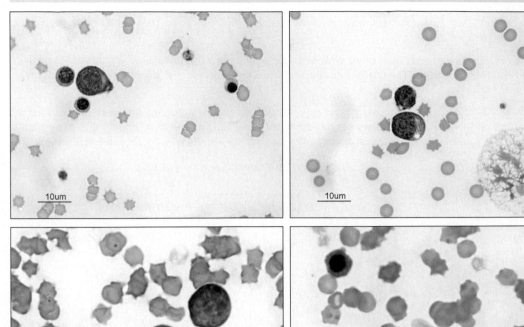

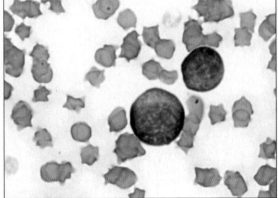

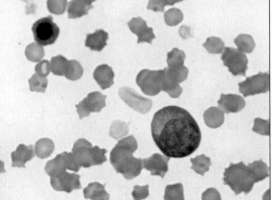

Acute Megakaryoblastic Leukemia

DISTINCTIVE FEATURES: Acute megakaryoblastic leukemia (AML-M7) is diagnosed on the basis of the presence of 20% or more blasts found in bone marrow, with 50% of these cells consistent with megakaryoblasts.

Megakaryoblasts are larger than other blast cells and may have a single nucleus or a lobulated nucleus from endomytotic divisions. The cytoplasm may be scant to moderate and often stains basophilic with cytoplasmic blebbing.

DIAGNOSTIC SIGNIFICANCE: Megakaryoblasts are extremely uncommon in the peripheral blood of normal dogs and cats. Although megakaryoblasts may have unique features, allowing differentiation from other myeloid blasts, cytochemistry and immunomarkers are often needed to define lineage.

Plate 5-5   Acute Megakaryoblastic Leukemia

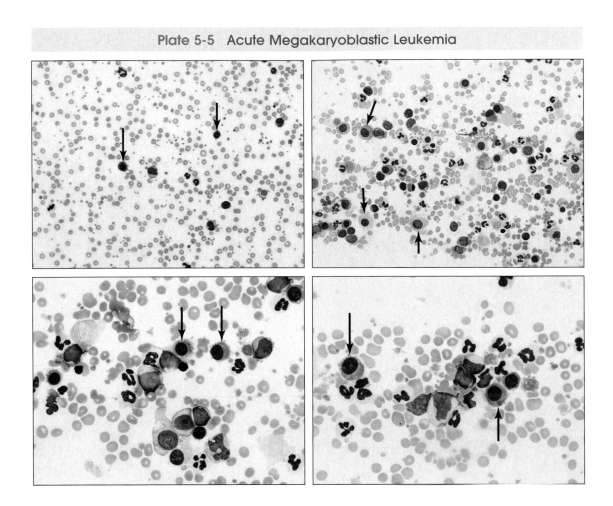

Plate 5-5   Acute Megakaryoblastic Leukemia *(con't)*

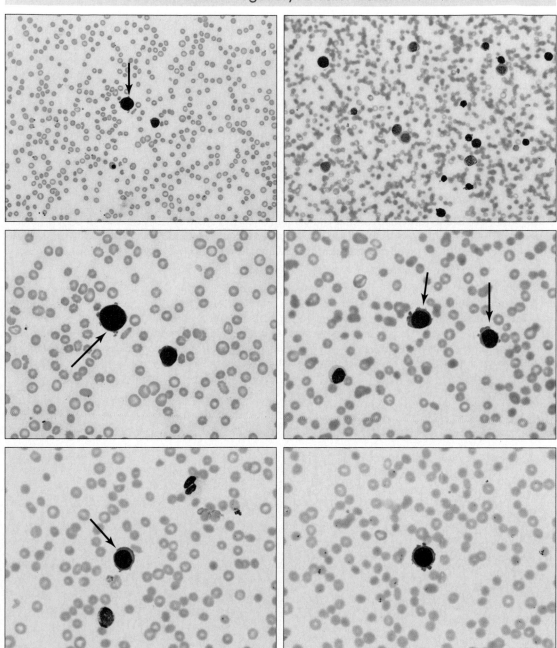

Chronic Myeloid Leukemia

All forms of chronic myelogenous leukemia are uncommon in dogs and cats and, when diagnosed, are most often a disease of older animals. The chronic leukemias are composed of mature, well-differentiated cells that are morphologically similar to their nonneoplastic counterparts. Diagnosis is based on finding large numbers of mature cells in peripheral blood that cannot be explained by underlying etiologies, which may be challenging at times. Often, serial CBC examinations are needed to document persistently high and, often, slowly increasing numbers of cells.

In contrast to acute leukemias, which consist of rapidly dividing blasts, which quickly efface the marrow and result in significant and often multiple cytopenias at the time of diagnosis, chronic leukemias are composed of mature, slowly developing and dividing cells. Thus, typically, cytopenias evolve only when high numbers of leukemic cells are present in peripheral blood.

Similar to chronic lymphocytic leukemia, monitoring of the CBC over time is needed to evaluate for an evolving blast crisis, signaling a transition from chronic leukemia to acute leukemia.

Chronic Granulocytic Leukemia

DISTINCTIVE FEATURES: Chronic granulocytic leukemia is diagnosed by the presence of large numbers of neutrophils, eosinophils, or basophils in peripheral blood and bone marrow. Mature forms predominate, with a left shift composed of lower numbers of immature forms (bands to myeloblasts). Dysplastic changes may be present.

DIAGNOSTIC SIGNIFICANCE: Chronic granulocytic leukemia may be difficult to distinguish from a severe neutrophilia or leukemoid response. Evidence of neutrophil toxic change (suggesting infection) and careful assessment of the patient for underlying inflammation, infection, and tissue necrosis, with close monitoring of the CBC over time, are helpful to differentiate the conditions. Chronic granulocytic leukemia may be associated with nonregenerative anemia and thrombocytopenia in the later stages of disease, when large numbers of circulating neoplastic cells are present.

Plate 5-6   Chronic Granulocytic Leukemia (Neutrophilic)

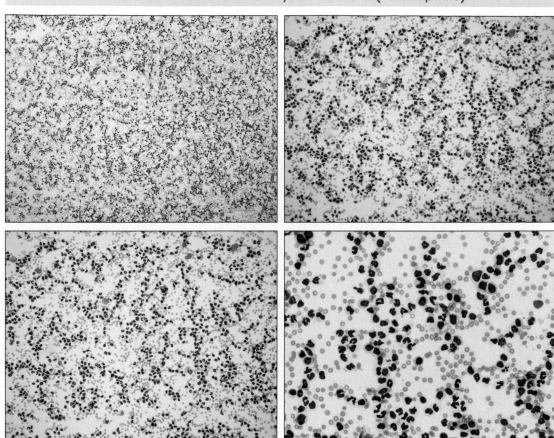

Plate 5-6 Chronic Granulocytic Leukemia (Neutrophilic) *(con't)*

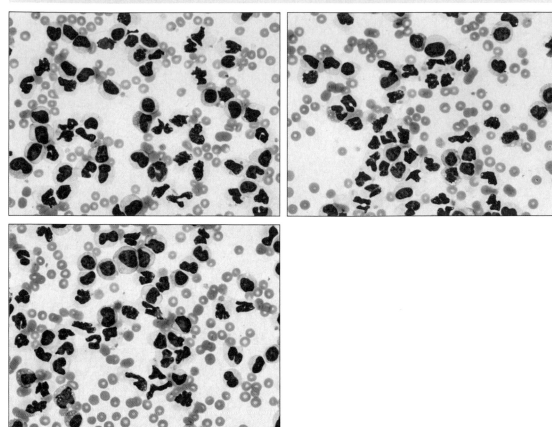

Plate 5-7   Chronic Granulocytic Leukemia (Eosinophilic)

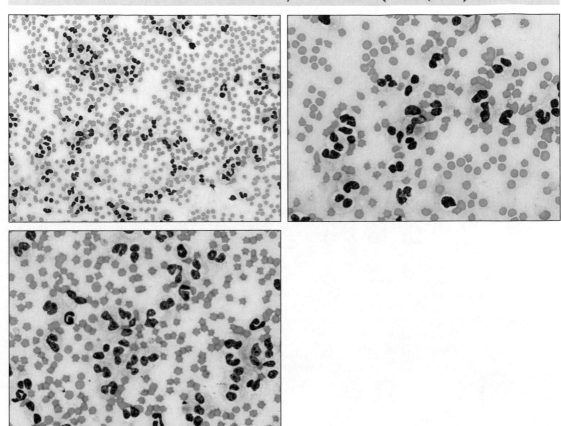

Chronic Monocytic Leukemia

DISTINCTIVE FEATURES: Chronic monocytic leukemia is diagnosed on the basis of large numbers of mature monocytes in peripheral blood and bone marrow. It may be associated with cytopenias in later stage of disease, when large numbers of circulating neoplastic cells are present.

Plate 5-8   Chronic Myeloid Leukemia (Monocytic)

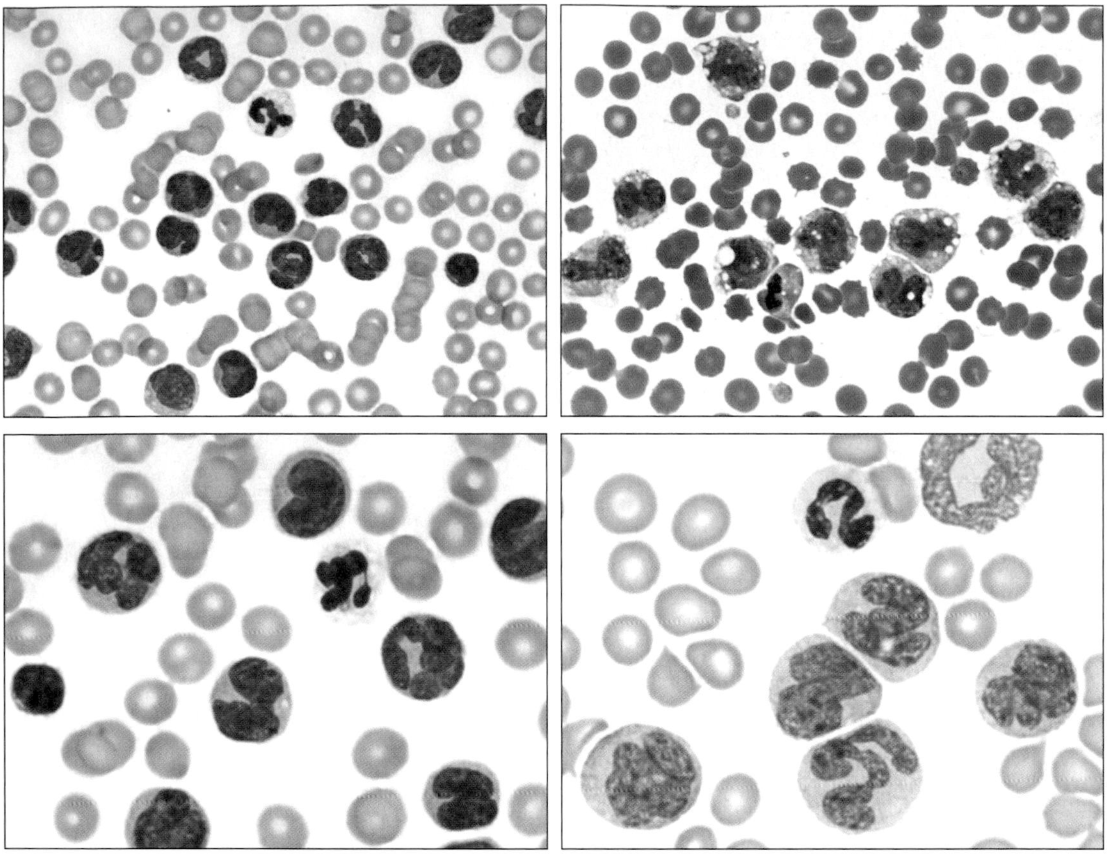

Plate 5-8   Chronic Myeloid Leukemia (Monocytic) *(con't)*

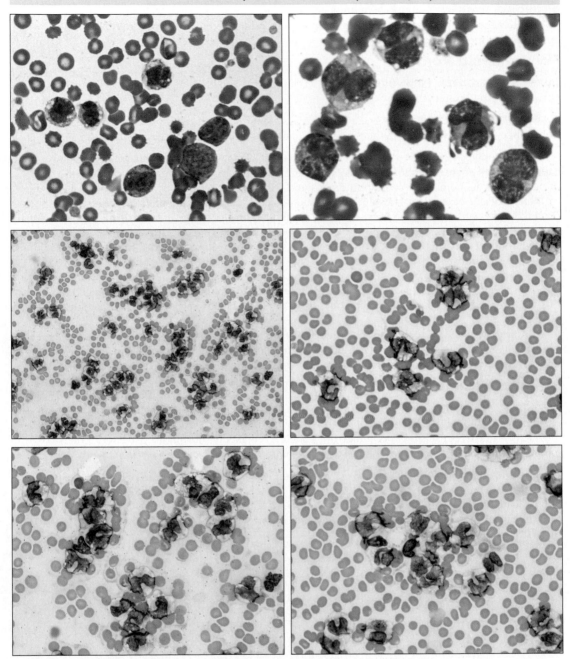

Chronic Myelomonocytic Leukemia

DISTINCTIVE FEATURES: Chronic myelomonocytic leukemia is diagnosed on the basis of large numbers of mature neutrophils and monocytes in peripheral blood and bone marrow. It may be associated with cytopenias in the later stages of disease.

Polycythemia Vera

DISTINCTIVE FEATURES: Polycythemia vera (PV) is a chronic leukemia of dogs and cats, in which persistent, unexplained polycythemia exists.

DIAGNOSTIC SIGNIFICANCE: Diagnosis of PV is based on excluding two much more common causes of polycythemia: (1) relative polycythemia and (2) nonneoplastic absolute polycythemia.

Relative polycythemia is secondary to dehydration or splenic contraction (catecholamine release caused by excitement). Dehydration may be determined by physical examination and by the presence of panhyperproteinemia or hyperalbuminemia and prerenal azotemia.

Nonneoplastic etiologies of absolute polycythemia may be appropriate physiologic responses such as production of erythropoietin (EPO) secondary to hypoxia from cardiac disease, respiratory disease, or both, resulting in an increase in RBC production. Assessment to rule out disease of the heart and lungs (auscultation of the thorax, thoracic radiography, ultrasonography, electrocardiography), blood gas assessment to confirm hypoxia, and measurement of EPO levels aid in diagnosis.

Inappropriate causes of absolute polycythemia are from increased EPO production in the absence of hypoxia, as in EPO-secreting neoplasms of the kidney or EPO secretion secondary to nonneoplastic renal disease. These are diagnosed when hypoxia is ruled out through blood gas assessment and measurement of EPO.

Additionally, some endocrinopathies such as hyperadrenocorticism (Cushing disease) and hyperthyroidism may result in polycythemia (hormonal stimulation of erythropoiesis) and may be diagnosed with a combination of serum chemistry tests, physical examination findings, and patient history.

Essential Thrombocythemia

DISTINCTIVE FEATURES: Essential thrombocythemia (ET) is a rare, chronic leukemia in dogs and cats. Diagnosis is based on the identification of sustained, chronic, unexplained, marked thrombocytosis with megakaryocytic hyperplasia of bone marrow. Platelets are usually normal in appearance but may be of variable size. Dysplastic changes and associated cytopenias are not commonly seen.

DIAGNOSTIC SIGNIFICANCE: Diagnosis of ET is based on excluding all causes of nonneoplastic thrombocytoses, the most common of which is a reactive thrombocytosis secondary to underlying inflammation, infection, neoplasia, and iron deficiency anemia. Other less common causes of a nonneoplastic thrombocytosis are secondary to certain drugs and splenic contraction (epinephrine release).

Additionally, thrombocytosis may also be seen with some forms of leukemia such as basophilic leukemia, PV, and acute megakaryoblastic leukemia.

Plate 5-9　Essential Thrombocythemia

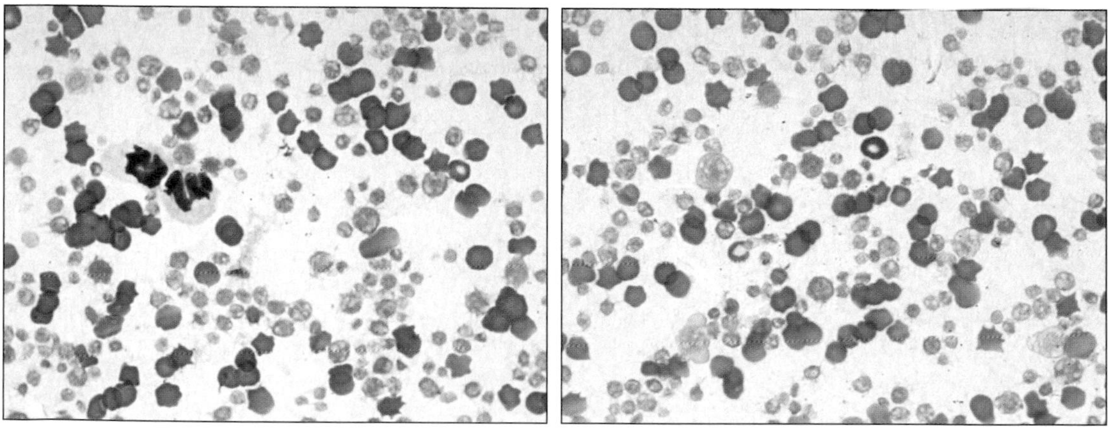

Plate 5-9 Essential Thrombocythemia *(con't)*

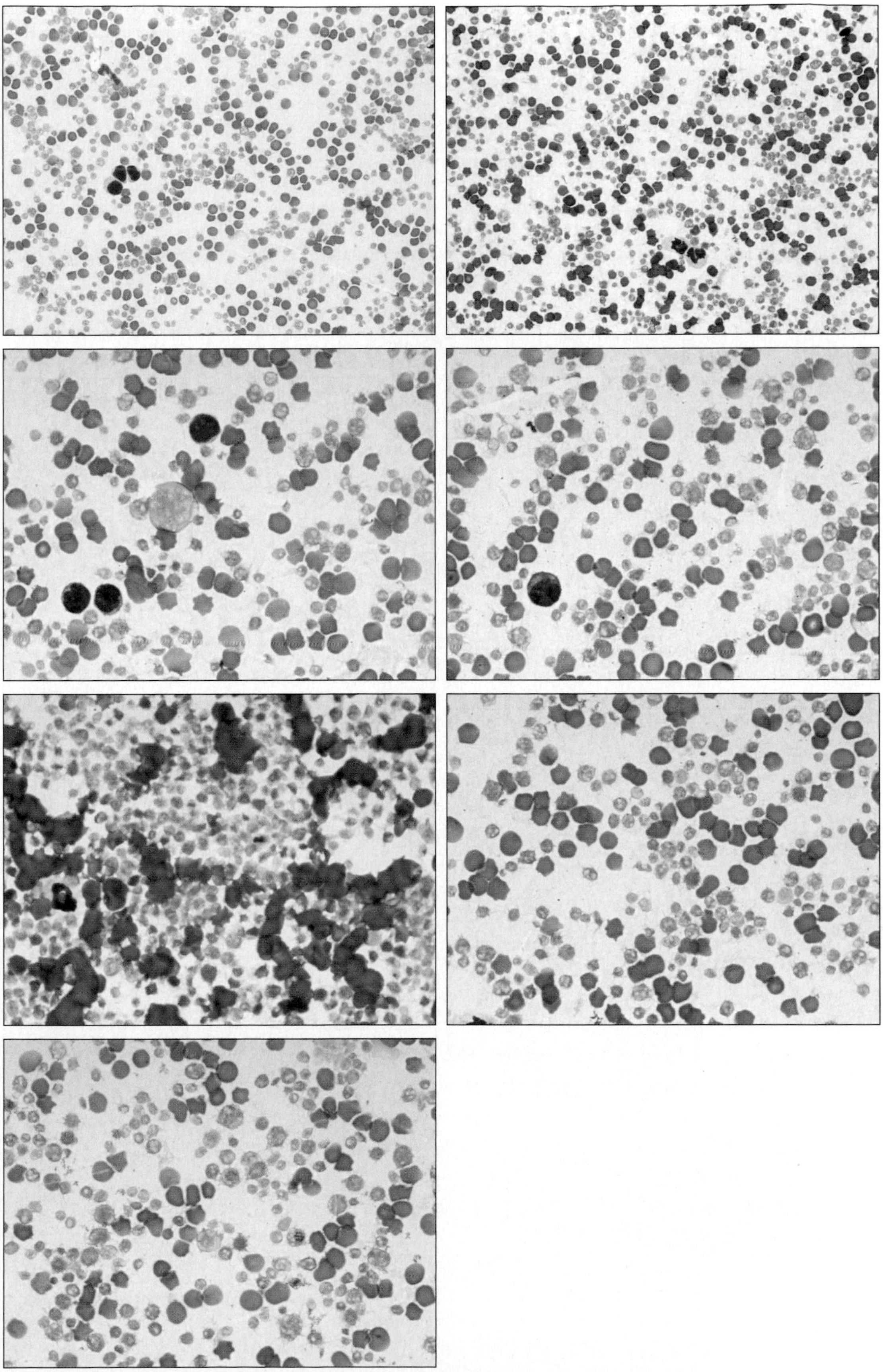

Mitotic Figures

DISTINCTIVE FEATURES: Mitotic figures are cells undergoing cell division. A well-defined nucleus is not seen; instead, chromatids are seen as dark purple (same color as the nucleus), linear structures forming a spindle. Mitotic cells may be found in any stage of mitoses, and thus, chromatids may be concentrated in the center of the cell, forming a spindle shape or pulled apart from the center and found in two polar groups. If the cell undergoing division is neoplastic, aberrant mitoses, in which the chromatids are dispersed randomly throughout the cytoplasm of the cell and appear disorganized, may be seen.

DIAGNOSTIC SIGNIFICANCE: Mitotic figures are not normally seen in the peripheral blood of normal dogs and cats. When present, they are often found at the feathered edges of the blood smear. Rarely, mitotic figures are seen in the peripheral blood of nonleukemic animals, in cases of reactive lymphocytosis, and rarely in cats with strongly regenerative anemias. Usually, when mitotic figures are found on peripheral blood smears, they are part of a leukemic cell population. Therefore, when mitotic figures are identified in peripheral blood smears, assessment for underlying leukemia is warranted.

Plate 5-10   Mitotic Figures

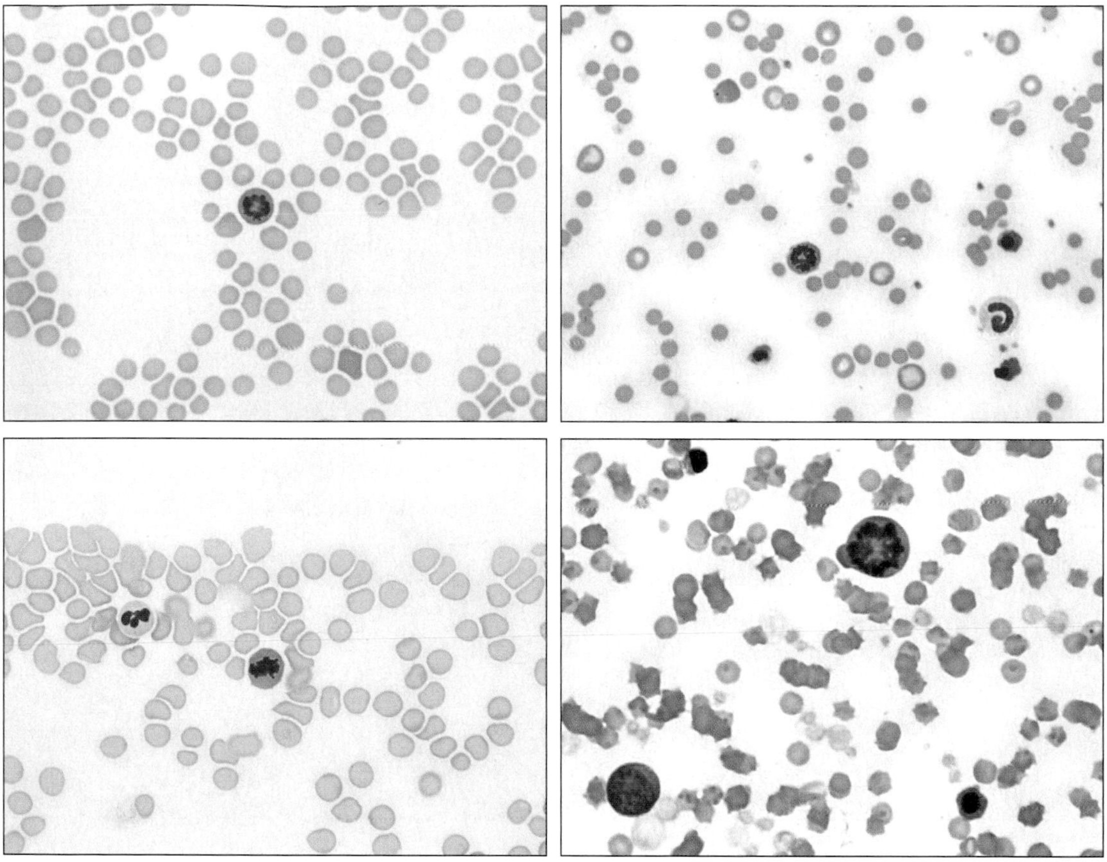

Plate 5-10   Mitotic Figures *(con't)*

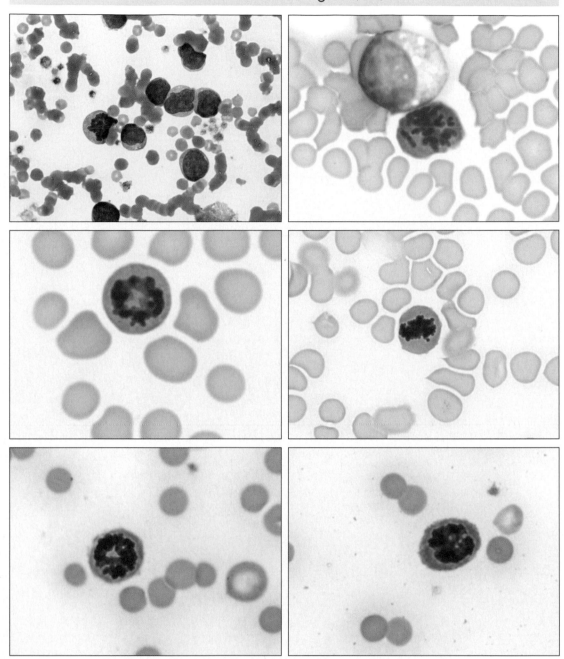

SECTION 6:
EXTRACELLULAR ORGANISMS

Microfilaria

DISTINCTIVE FEATURES: Microfilariae from *Dirofilaria immitis* or *Acanthocheilonema reconditum* (*Dipetalonema reconditum*) are large, extracellular filarial larvae, which have an elongated "wormlike" body. In general, *D. immitis* (L1) larvae are usually present in high numbers, have a stationary or nonprogressive movement in wet preps, a straight body, a straight tail, and a tapered head. In contrast, *A. reconditum* larvae generally are few in number, have a progressive movement in wet preps, a curved body, and a blunt head. Differentiation based on microscopic evaluation is difficult, and mixed infections may occur.

DIAGNOSTIC SIGNIFICANCE: The presence of filarial larvae indicates infection with either or both *D. immitis* or *A. reconditum.*

Plate 6-1   Microfilaria

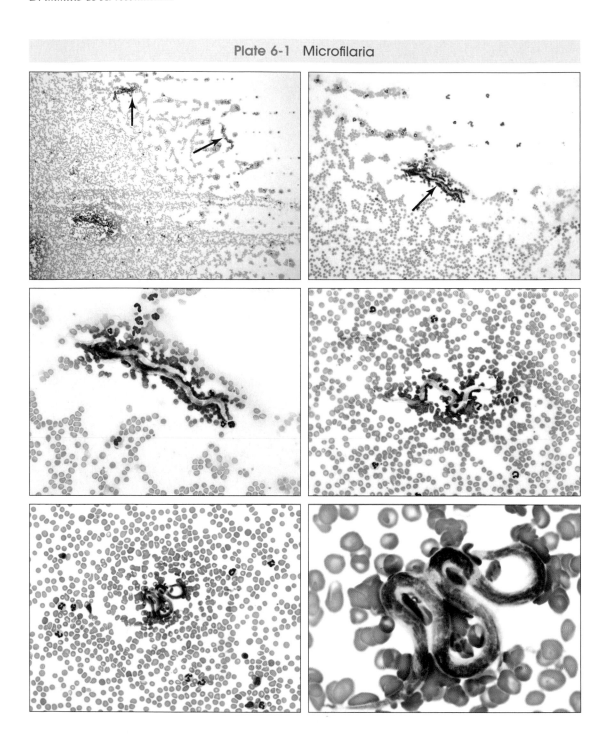

Plate 6-1 Microfilaria *(con't)*

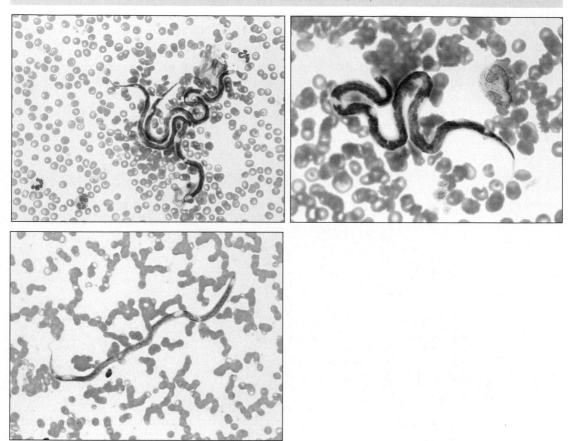

A, Fibrin strand **B,** Two microfilaria

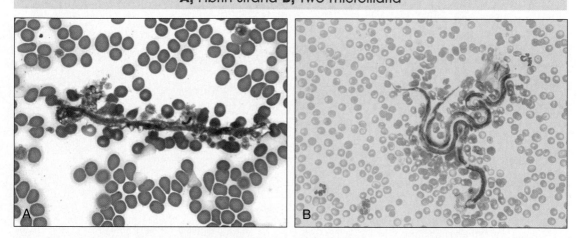

Trypanosomes

DISTINCTIVE FEATURES: Trypomastigotes, the flagellated stage of trypanosomes found in peripheral blood, are large, extracellular protozoa that have an elongated or "blade-shaped" body with an undulating membrane, a tapering posterior end, and a short flagellum directed anteriorly.

DIAGNOSTIC SIGNIFICANCE: The presence of trypanosomes in peripheral blood indicates trypanosomiasis. Trypanosomiasis is a zoonotic disease, and dogs and cats are important reservoirs of infection. In the United States, trypanosomal infection is most often caused by *Trypanosoma cruzi* (Chagas disease) and is transmitted by biting triatomine bugs, resulting in systemic infection and many variable clinical signs. The predominant clinical manifestation is cardiac disease secondary to myocarditis.

Plate 6-2 Trypanosomes

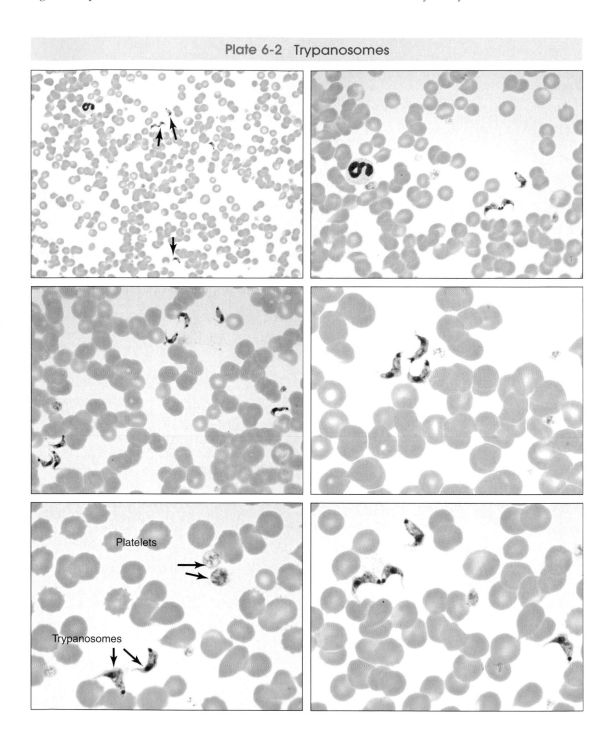

Plate 6-2 Trypanosomes *(con't)*

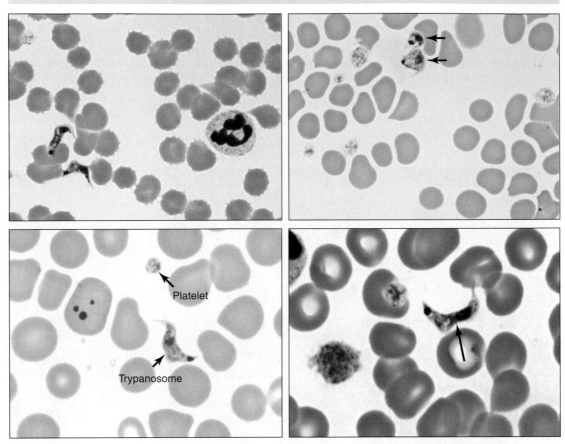

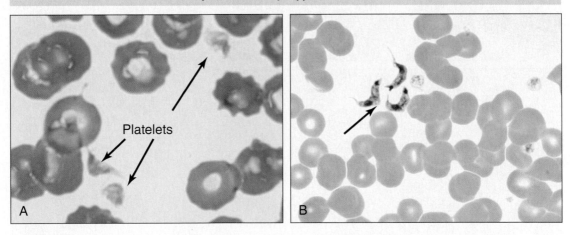

Make sure not to confuse curve shaped platelets with trypanosomes.
A, Platelets **B,** Trypanosomes

Spirochetes

DISTINCTIVE FEATURES: Spirochetes are rarely seen in peripheral blood and are bacteria of the order *Spirochaetales*. Spirochetes appear as small, thin, corkscrew-shaped, extracellular organisms.

DIAGNOSTIC SIGNIFICANCE: The presence of spirochetes in peripheral blood suggests borreliosis or lyme disease, which is a tickborne disease caused by the bacterium *Borrelia burgdorferi*. Finding spirochetes on peripheral blood films warrants further testing, empirical antibiotic therapy, or both.

Plate 6-3   Spirochetes

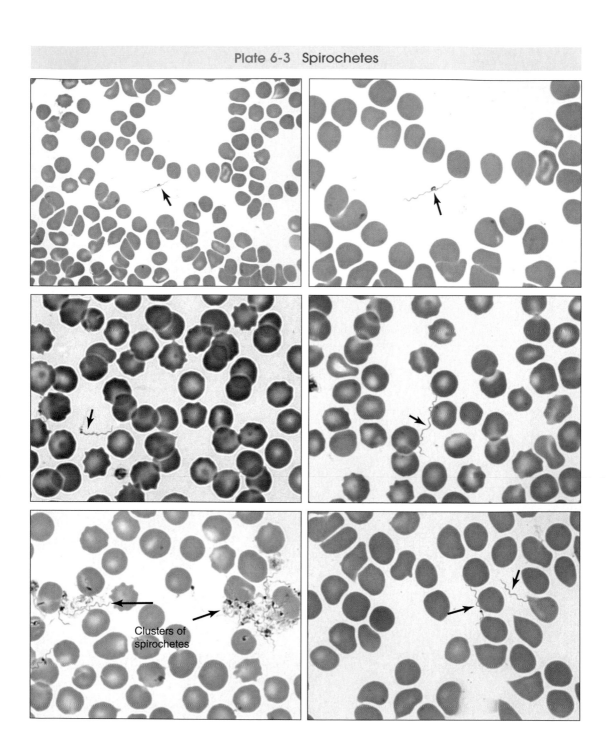

Clusters of
spirochetes

Plate 6-3 Spirochetes *(con't)*

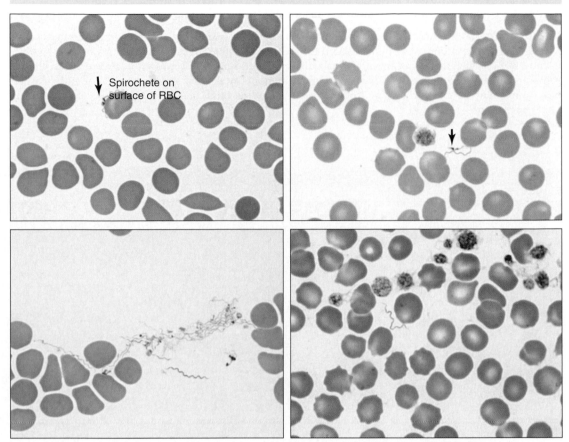

Spirochete on surface of RBC

Make sure not to confuse activated platelets with spirochetes and platelet fragments. A, Activated Platelet **B,** Platelet Fragment **C,** Spriochetes

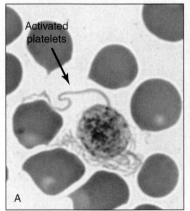

Activated platelets

A

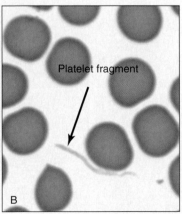

Platelet fragment

B

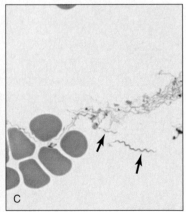

C

Bacteria

DISTINCTIVE FEATURES: Moderate numbers of extracellular bacterial rods or cocci may occur.

DIAGNOSTIC SIGNIFICANCE: Bacterial overgrowth occurs occasionally in ethylenediaminetetraacetic acid (EDTA) tubes and must be differentiated from true septicemia. Bacterial septicemia usually has low numbers of intracellular organisms and markedly toxic neutrophils and must be correlated with clinical signs and history of the patient. Bacterial contamination usually has only extracellular bacteria (the neutrophils may be toxic or have no toxic change, depending on the health status of the patient during blood sampling).

Plate 6-4   Extracellular Bacteria

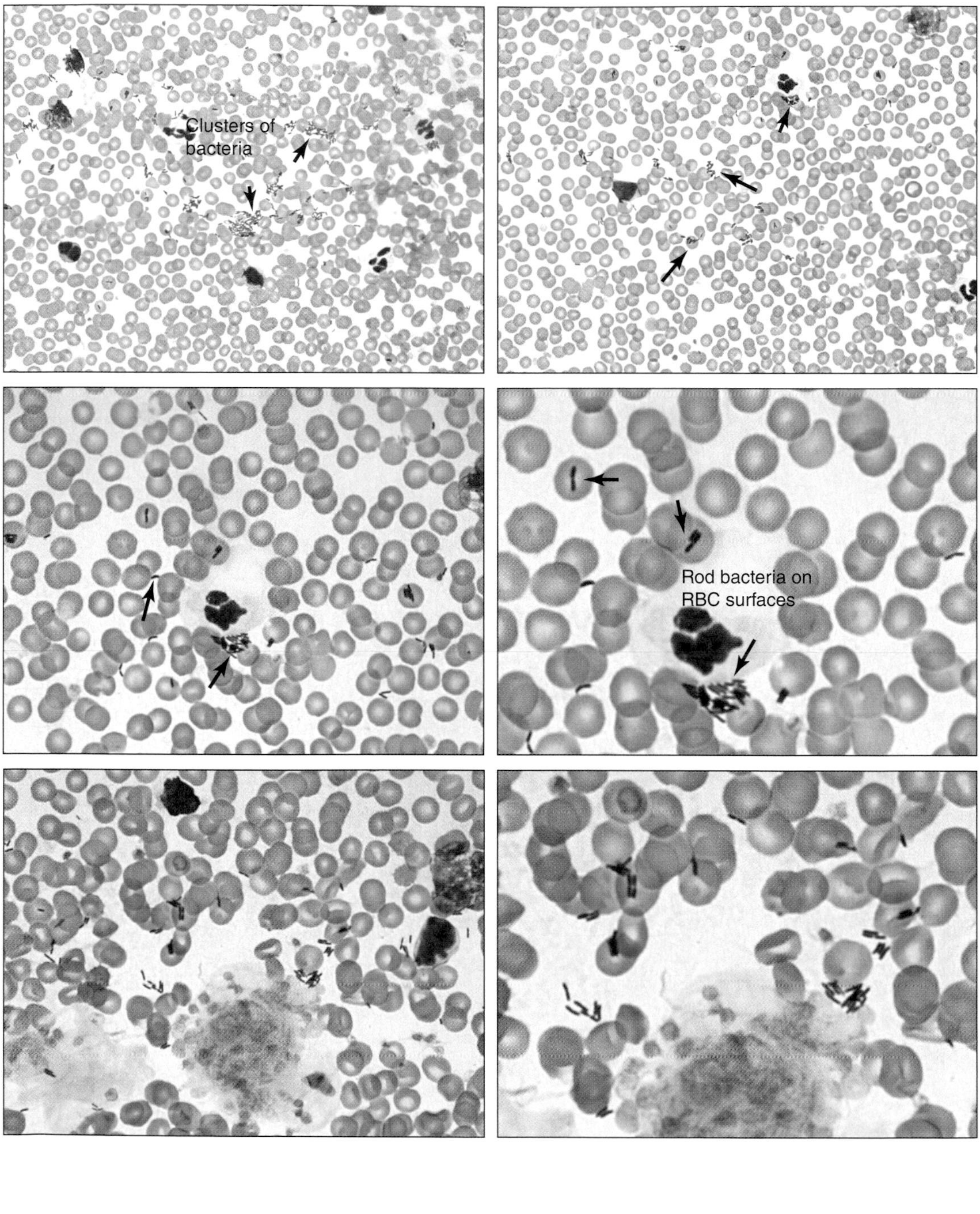

Plate 6-4 Extracellular Bacteria *(con't)*

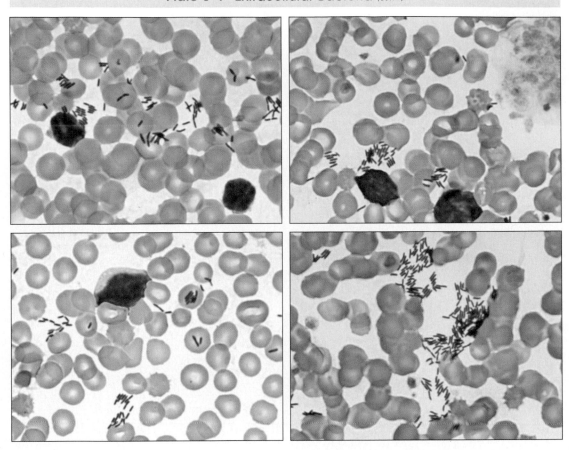

Make sure to distinguish bacteria (rare) from clumps of stain precipitant (common). **A,** Stain precipitation. Note globular to amorphous appearance **B,** Bacteria. Note distinct uniform rod shape

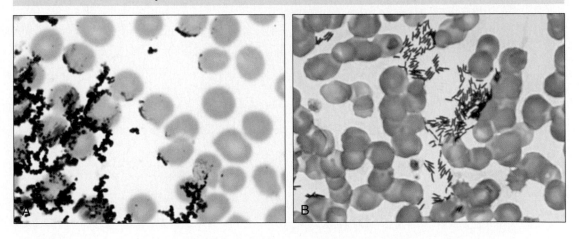

Plate 6-1   Microfilaria *(con't)*

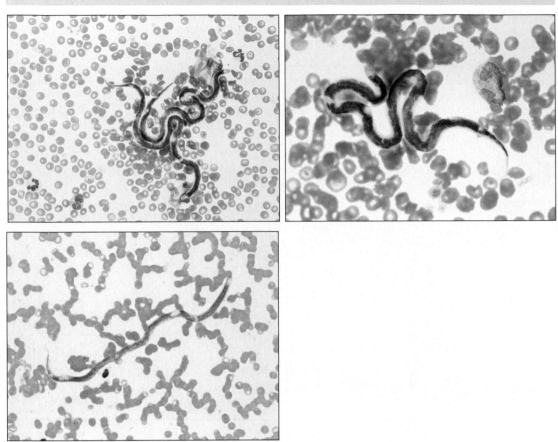

A, Fibrin strand **B,** Two microfilaria

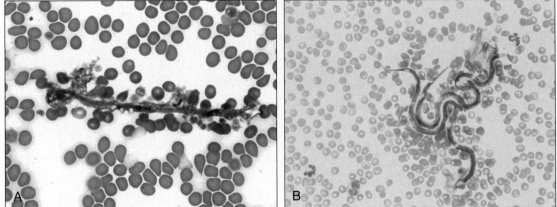

Trypanosomes

DISTINCTIVE FEATURES: Trypomastigotes, the flagellated stage of trypanosomes found in peripheral blood, are large, extracellular protozoa that have an elongated or "blade-shaped" body with an undulating membrane, a tapering posterior end, and a short flagellum directed anteriorly.

DIAGNOSTIC SIGNIFICANCE: The presence of trypanosomes in peripheral blood indicates trypanosomiasis. Trypanosomiasis is a zoonotic disease, and dogs and cats are important reservoirs of infection. In the United States, trypanosomal infection is most often caused by *Trypanosoma cruzi* (Chagas disease) and is transmitted by biting triatomine bugs, resulting in systemic infection and many variable clinical signs. The predominant clinical manifestation is cardiac disease secondary to myocarditis.

Plate 6-2 Trypanosomes

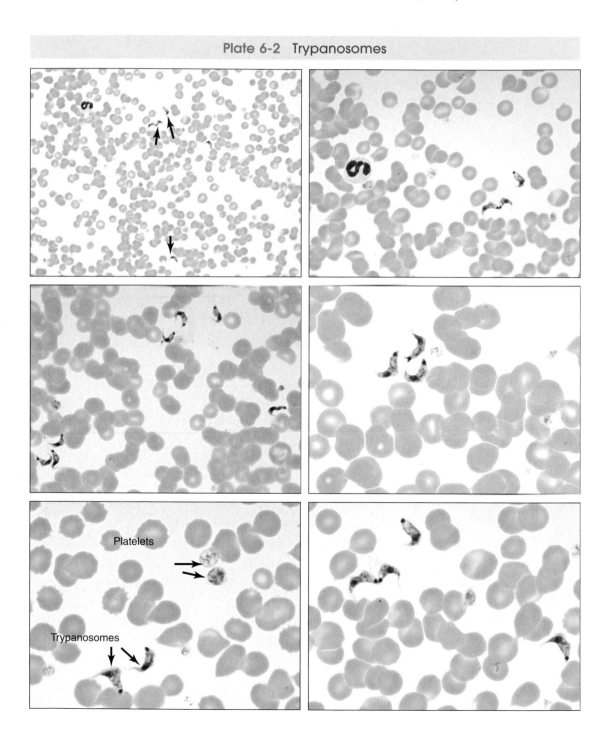

Plate 6-2 Trypanosomes *(con't)*

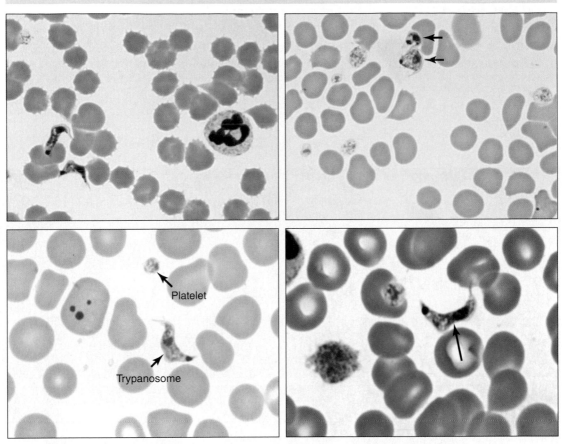

Make sure not to confuse curve shaped platelets with trypanosomes.
A, Platelets **B,** Trypanosomes

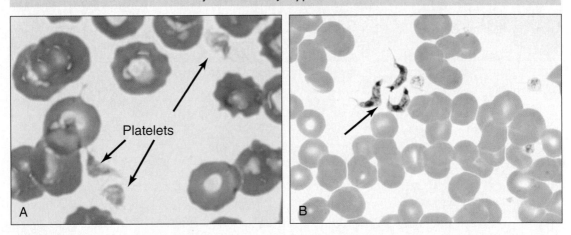

Spirochetes

DISTINCTIVE FEATURES: Spirochetes are rarely seen in peripheral blood and are bacteria of the order *Spirochaetales*. Spirochetes appear as small, thin, corkscrew-shaped, extracellular organisms.

DIAGNOSTIC SIGNIFICANCE: The presence of spirochetes in peripheral blood suggests borreliosis or lyme disease, which is a tickborne disease caused by the bacterium *Borrelia burgdorferi*. Finding spirochetes on peripheral blood films warrants further testing, empirical antibiotic therapy, or both.

Plate 6-3   Spirochetes

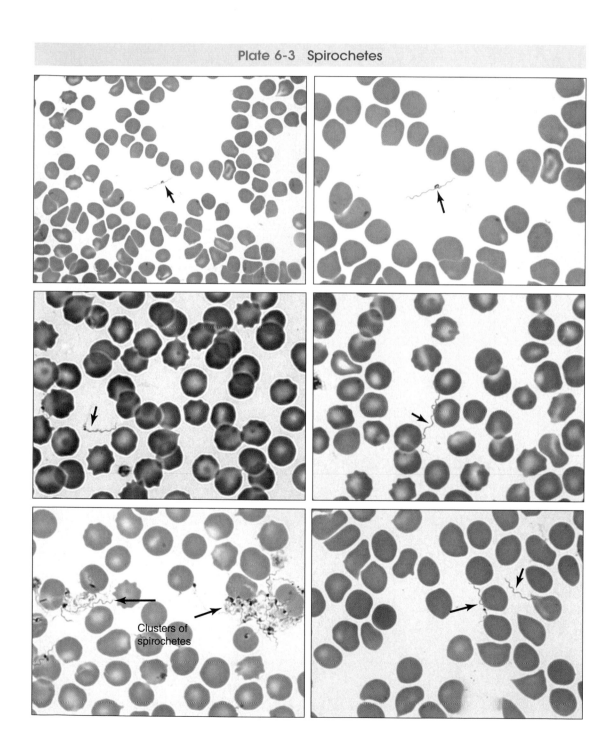

Clusters of spirochetes

Plate 6-3   Spirochetes *(con't)*

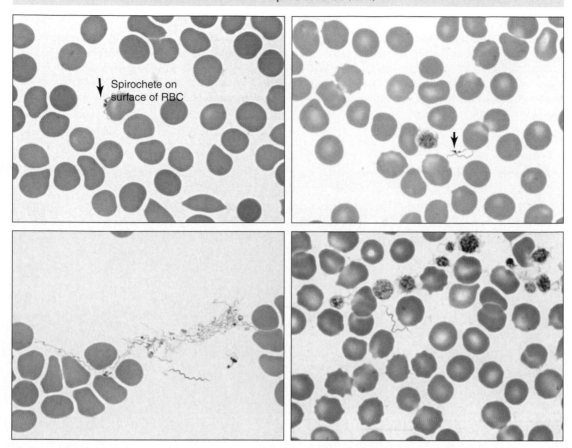

Spirochete on surface of RBC

Make sure not to confuse activated platelets with spirochetes and platelet fragments. **A,** Activated Platelet **B,** Platelet Fragment **C,** Spriochetes

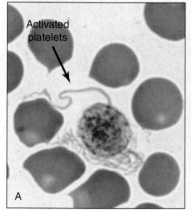

Activated platelets

A

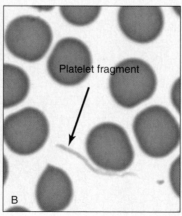

Platelet fragment

B

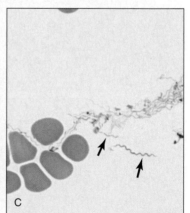

C

Bacteria

DISTINCTIVE FEATURES: Moderate numbers of extracellular bacterial rods or cocci may occur.

DIAGNOSTIC SIGNIFICANCE: Bacterial overgrowth occurs occasionally in ethylenediaminetetraacetic acid (EDTA) tubes and must be differentiated from true septicemia. Bacterial septicemia usually has low numbers of intracellular organisms and markedly toxic neutrophils and must be correlated with clinical signs and history of the patient. Bacterial contamination usually has only extracellular bacteria (the neutrophils may be toxic or have no toxic change, depending on the health status of the patient during blood sampling).

Plate 6-4   Extracellular Bacteria

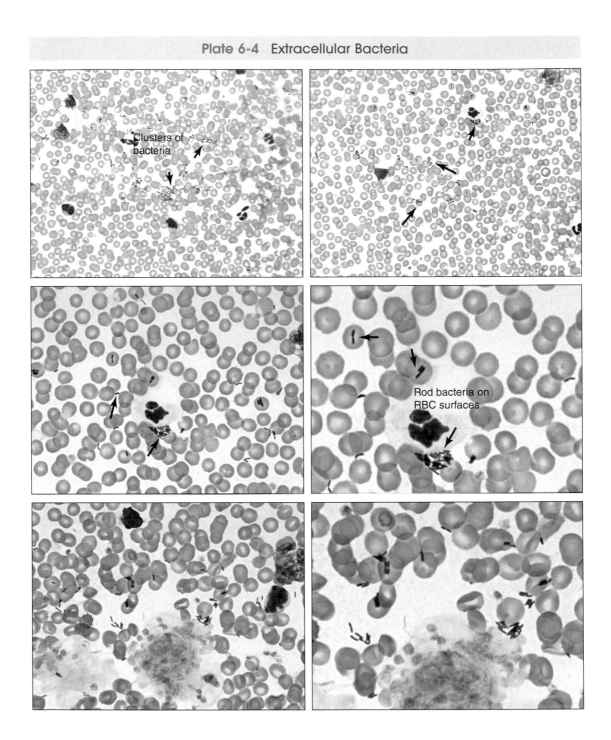

Plate 6-4   Extracellular Bacteria *(con't)*

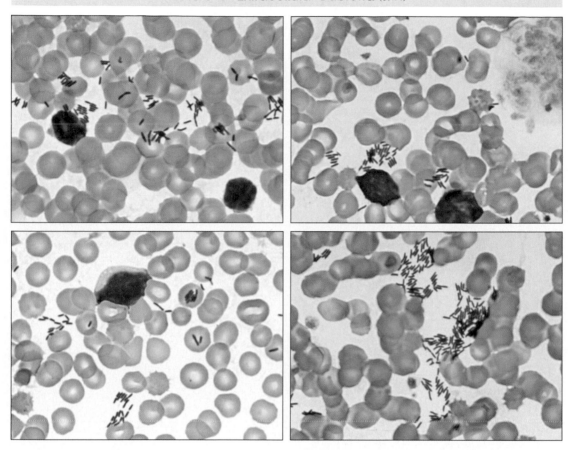

Make sure to distinguish bacteria (rare) from clumps of stain precipitant (common). **A,** Stain precipitation. Note globular to amorphous appearance **B,** Bacteria. Note distinct uniform rod shape

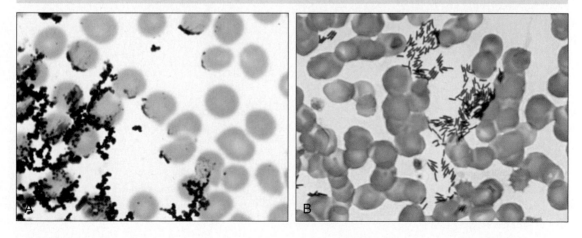

APPENDIX

Reticulocyte Count

The reticulocyte count, which is used to assess bone marrow response to anemia, is a more sensitive measurement of bone marrow regenerative response than is polychromasia because a greater concentration of ribosomes in red blood cell (RBC) cytoplasm is required for RBCs to stain polychromatophilic with Romanowsky-type (Wright) stains than is required for RBC to stain as reticulocytes with supravital stains (new methylene blue [NMB]). Thus, all polychromatophilic cells stain as reticulocytes with supravital stains, whereas some reticulocytes do not stain polychromatophilic with Romanowsky-type stains. The reticulocyte count may be performed in-house or by referral laboratories. Box 1 gives the procedure for performing in-house reticulocyte counts. Referral laboratories may perform reticulocyte counts on ethylenediaminetetraacetic acid (EDTA) blood samples submitted for hemogram analysis or for other reasons. Relative reticulocyte counts are reported as the percentage of RBCs that are reticulocytes. Absolute reticulocyte counts are reported as the number of reticulocytes per volume of blood. When possible, the absolute reticulocyte count should be used to evaluate the regenerative response rather than the relative reticulocyte count.

Reticulocytes are young RBCs containing a sufficient concentration of polyribosomes so that after incubation in supravital stains such as NMB, polyribosomes aggregate forming blue-black dots or aggregates. Reticulocytes do not increase to what is considered adequate levels to immediately classify an anemia as regenerative. It takes approximately 2 days for the number of young RBCs to increase in the circulation and 5 to 7 days for them to reach a maximum level with most acute anemias that are

---

BOX 1   New Methylene Blue Stain for Reticulocytes

A. Principle
New methylene blue is a cationic dye capable of penetrating the living cell and precipitating the ribosomes of the immature red blood cell (RBC). In the reticulocyte, new methylene blue (NMB) stain precipitates with the remnants of the endoplasmic reticulum (ER), which is primarily the ribosome and messenger ribonucleic acid (mRNA) for hemoglobin synthesis. As the RBC matures, the ER is lost, so only cells recently released from bone marrow into the circulation will contain the ER. Therefore, the reticulocyte count estimates the bone marrow response to anemia.

B. Procedure
1. Place equal amounts of NMB stain and ethylenediaminetetraacetic acid (EDTA) blood in a test tube for 20 minutes.
2. From this mixture, make a blood smear.
3. Count 1000 RBCs, recording the number of reticulocytes observed in these 1000 cells.

C. Calculation of Reticulocyte Count

$$\frac{\text{number of reticulocytes counted per 1000 RBC}}{10} = \%\ \text{reticulocytes}$$

regenerative (hemorrhage or hemolysis). Therefore, an acute anemia may appear nonregenerative by a reticulocyte count performed before young RBCs have increased in the circulation.

In dogs and cats, the reticulocyte count increases proportionately to the severity of anemia if the anemia is regenerative (i.e., bone marrow regeneration is occurring appropriately in response to the anemia). As erythropoiesis increases in response to anemia, young RBCs are released into the circulation 1 to 2 days earlier than normal. As a result, they are within the circulation but still stainable as reticulocytes for 1 or 2 days longer than under normal conditions. Also, the increase in erythropoiesis causes many more young RBCs to be produced and released. Hence, increased erythropoiesis is accompanied by an increase in peripheral blood reticulocyte count proportional to the magnitude of increased erythropoiesis, which is, in turn, proportional to the severity of anemia.

In cats, reticulocytes may be divided into two morphologic classes: (1) punctate reticulocytes and (2) aggregate reticulocytes. Punctate reticulocytes are RBCs containing a few small, dotlike (punctate), blue-black structures (small polyribosome aggregates) but no large aggregates of ribosomes. Aggregate reticulocytes are RBCs containing one or more medium to large, blue-black structures that may appear as a cluster or network of aggregated structures. Punctate and aggregate reticulocytes should be differentiated and counted separately. Counting the number of punctate reticulocytes may be very time consuming, as they can reach very high numbers. Therefore, in moderate to severe anemias, punctate reticulocytes are frequently not counted, since bone marrow regenerative response is interpreted solely on the basis of aggregate reticulocyte numbers in moderate to severe anemias.

Feline punctate reticulocytes represent a later maturational stage of feline aggregate reticulocytes. The feline aggregate reticulocyte circulates only about 1 day before sufficient ribosomes are degraded for it to stain as a punctate reticulocyte. Feline aggregate reticulocyte counts are interpreted similarly to reticulocyte counts in dogs and cattle. However, in mild anemias, feline aggregate reticulocytes may be held in bone marrow until they reach the punctate stage, resulting in little or no increase in peripheral blood aggregate reticulocyte numbers. Feline punctate reticulocytes may occur in high numbers (up to 10%) in health, increase during regenerative anemia, and may be elevated during mild regenerative anemia without concurrent elevation of feline aggregate reticulocytes. Also, punctate reticulocytes may be elevated during severe nonregenerative or poorly regenerative anemias without an appropriate concurrent elevation of feline aggregate reticulocytes. Because feline punctate reticulocytes may be increased during mild anemia without concurrent increase in feline aggregate reticulocytes, feline punctate reticulocytes may be helpful in determining whether mild anemias are regenerative or nonregenerative. For example, high numbers of punctate reticulocytes in a cat with mild anemia of sufficient duration to allow bone marrow response suggests regenerative anemia, even if the aggregate reticulocyte count is not increased. Whereas, an absence of an increase in punctate reticulocytes in the peripheral blood of a cat with mild anemia of sufficient duration to allow bone marrow response suggests nonregenerative anemia unless an increase in aggregate reticulocytes occurs. In cats, an increase in the aggregate reticulocytes without concurrent increase in punctate reticulocytes suggests early bone marrow response to anemia. In a few days, the increased numbers of aggregate reticulocytes will mature, causing an increase in punctate reticulocyte numbers. Cats with moderate to severe anemia of sufficient duration to allow bone marrow response should have an increased aggregate reticulocyte count. If they do not, the anemia is very likely nonregenerative or poorly regenerative regardless of the punctate reticulocyte count. For example, a cat that has had a packed cell volume (PCV) of 10 for a week and has an aggregate reticulocyte count of 0.1% and a punctate reticulocyte count of 25% has a nonregenerative anemia. If punctate reticulocytes are counted as aggregate reticulocytes, nonregenerative or poorly regenerative anemias may be misclassified as regenerative anemias; however, failure to count punctate reticulocytes may cause some adequately regenerative mild anemias to be misclassified as inadequately regenerative.

Absolute Reticulocyte Count

The absolute reticulocyte count is the number of reticulocytes per microliter (reticulocytes/µL) of blood. The absolute reticulocyte count more accurately reflects the bone marrow's response compared with the percent reticulocyte count because it automatically adjusts for the decrease in mature RBC numbers, preventing a misimpression of increase in reticulocytes that may be given by percent reticulocyte count during anemia. For example, a dog that normally has a PCV of 40%, an RBC count of 6,000,000 reticulocytes/µL, and a percent reticulocyte count of 1% would have an absolute reticulocyte count of 60,000/µL (1% of 6,000,000 = 60,000). If the dog becomes severely anemic with the hematocrit (HCT) and RBC count dropping to one fourth of the original values (10 and 1,500,000 reticulocytes/µL, respectively), a reticulocyte count of 3% would appear to indicate increased bone marrow reticulocyte production, when, in reality, a 3% reticulocyte count with a 1,500,000/µL RBC count represents only 45,000 reticulocytes/µL. Hence, although the percent reticulocyte count was increased, the actual number of

---

BOX 2   Calculations for Determining the Basal Reticulocyte Production Rate

A. The basal reticulocyte production rate (BRPR) is used to make adjustments for decreased sequestration of reticulocytes and increased pore size of marrow endothelial cells during anemia and to adjust for the decreased number of mature erythrocytes present during anemia.
   1. Basal production rate is useful in dogs only.
   2. Basal production rate greater than 1 is considered a responding anemia.
B. Calculation of BRPR:

$$\text{reticulocyte coun} \times \frac{\text{observed packed cell volume (PCV)}}{\substack{\text{normal PCV} \\ \text{(usually considered} \\ \text{to be 40)}}} \times \frac{1}{\substack{\text{correction factor} \\ \text{[see below]}}} = \text{BRPR}$$

C. Correction factors for the various hematocrit (HCT) values are given below:

HCT	Correction Factor
≥35%	1.0
25–35%	1.5
15–25%	2.0
≤15%	2.5

D. Sample calculation of BRPR for a dog with an HCT of 10% and a reticulocyte count of 15%:

$$15 \times \frac{10}{40} \times \frac{1}{2.5} = 15 \times 0.25 \times 0.4 = 1.5 \text{ BRPR}$$

---

reticulocytes in peripheral blood was decreased, indicating a nonregenerative, or poorly regenerative, anemia.

Basal Reticulocyte Production Rate

In dogs, a basal reticulocyte production rate (BRPR) has been determined empirically and may be particularly useful for evaluating a regenerative response when only HCT and percent reticulocytes are known. The BRPR adjusts for the decrease in numbers of mature RBCs, the increased time that reticulocytes circulate as reticulocytes because of their early release from bone marrow during anemia, and the expected proportional increase in erythropoiesis as the severity of anemia increases. To determine the BRPR, the patient's percent reticulocyte count is multiplied by the patient's actual HCT divided by the patient's expected normal HCT (usually predicted as 40), and the resulting value is divided by the appropriate BRPR correction factor. BRPRs above 1 indicate adequate bone marrow response to the anemia, whereas those less than 1 indicate inadequate bone marrow response to the anemia. Thus far, BRPR correction factors have been determined only for dogs. The formula and the correction factors used for calculating the BRPR are given in Box 2 along with a sample calculation.

Saline Dilution or Dispersion Test

RBC autoagglutination and rouleaux formation may be differentiated by saline dilution. Saline dilution may be performed by mixing equal amounts of physiologic saline and EDTA-anticoagulated blood, placing a drop of the mixture on a microscope slide, then placing a coverslip over the saline–blood mixture, and examining the unstained mixture microscopically for clumping. If the clumping is caused by autoagglutination, cell clumps will persist after saline dilution, and an unorganized or random (agglutinated) association of RBCs will be recognized. If clumping is caused by rouleaux formation, the cells will either disperse into individual cells, or an organized side-to-side rouleaux pattern (resembling a roll of coins) will easily be recognized.

INDEX

Page numbers followed by "f" indicate figures, "t" indicate tables, and "b" indicate boxes.